Sarah Ahrens et al. (eds.)
Accessibility – Health Literacy – Health Information

Silvia Hansen-Schirra / Christiane Maaß (eds.)
Easy – Plain – Accessible
Vol. 13

Sarah Ahrens/Rebecca Schulz/Janina Kröger/
Sergio Hernández Garrido/Loraine Keller/Isabel Rink (eds.)

Accessibility – Health Literacy – Health Information

Interdisciplinary Approaches to an Emerging Field of Communication

Frank & Timme
Verlag für wissenschaftliche Literatur

ISBN 978-3-7329-0895-0
ISBN E-Book 978-3-7329-9109-9
ISSN 2699-1683

Herstellung durch Frank & Timme GmbH,
Wittelsbacherstraße 27a, 10707 Berlin.
Printed in Germany.
Gedruckt auf säurefreiem, alterungsbeständigem Papier.

www.frank-timme.de

Contents

Ansgar Jonietz

Preface

It is hard to imagine a time before the term 'health literacy' was coined, as it is one of the most frequently discussed topics in the healthcare sector. But that was not always the case. The term essentially did not even exist a few years ago – at least not online. Google Trends lists the popularity of 'Health Literacy' as well as the German word 'Gesundheitskompetenz' as zero in January 2011, which was when I first started to deal with the topic of comprehensible healthcare information for patients. Even at that time, patients expressed a great desire for comprehensible information. However, this need was rarely met. The extent of associated health-related consequences for individuals and the healthcare system as a whole was still largely underestimated at that time. But a lot has happened since then. There are now more than 400 million search results on Google for 'Health Literacy' and there were over 3,500 entries in the Pubmed library alone in 2021. Major health literacy studies in recent years have certainly contributed to this increase. They revealed that many people have significant problems finding, understanding and properly applying good health information. In Germany, the results were even worse than the European average.

In parallel with the scientific findings, it also became increasingly clear that something had changed in the daily lives of the major players in the healthcare system: patients have long wanted to play a more prominent role in the decision-making process; at the same time they no longer rely solely on the expertise of medical contacts, but instead seek information on the internet. Unfortunately, 'Dr Google' is not a licensed doctor, but instead a mix of emotionally tinted lay reports, biased websites of profit-based companies, technically correct but incomprehensible information for those who are not medical professionals mixed in with what searchers actually need: evidence-based, independent, comprehensible and easily accessible information. The online jungle can make health literacy much more difficult. Therefore, health literacy is more important than ever before in our times of constant access to disorganised information.

Solutions that focus on health literacy are urgently needed at all points in the patient journey. The lack of accessible, comprehensible and individually tailored health information is still an acute problem. Patient-friendly health information is fundamental, regardless of whether it is used when people are googling symptoms, searching for a doctor, or talking to a doctor; or when doctors are informing patients before interventions; or to help understand findings, discharge reports, and all other documents that patients receive. Of course, this also applies to all information related to preventive measures and health-promoting behaviour. Even healthy people need good information that they can easily understand in order to stay healthy.

With the combined knowledge of medicine, communication and information technology, barrier-free access to comprehensible information can become standard procedure. But this is only possible if comprehensible information for patients becomes a permanent fixture in everyday healthcare, because comprehensibility has been proven to promote health literacy. The new awareness of health literacy and the importance of easily accessible, comprehensible health information go hand-in-hand with the realisation that changes in practice are urgently needed. Good organizational health literacy can compensate for low health literacy at the personal level. The current state of research already shows ways in which relatively simple solutions can have a measurable impact on patients' health literacy. However, much research is still needed to make health literacy an integral part of the healthcare system in the long term. This can be achieved only through barrier-free access to good health information. This volume illustrates the significance of this topic today and identifies the current insights and approaches to dealing with it.

Sarah Ahrens / Rebecca Schulz / Janina Kröger / Sergio Hernández Garrido / Loraine Keller / Isabel Rink

Accessible Communication and Health Literacy

1 Introduction

As more than half of the people in Germany describe experiencing difficulties in finding, understanding, appraising and applying health information (Schaeffer et al. 2021: 26), the need for comprehensible and appropriate health-related information is growing tremendously. Especially people with a low socioeconomic status, low level of education and people over the age of 65 are affected by low health literacy (ibid. 28). Being chronically ill, having a communication impairment, a low socioeconomic status and/or non-native background (Schaeffer et al. 2016: 41) can inhibit the successful reception of health information which can increase health inequalities and obstruct participation. Vulnerable target groups in particular (e.g. people with cognitive or sensory impairments, or of old age) face distinct barriers in the use of health information. The target groups of accessible communication coincide with the vulnerable groups mentioned in the National Action Plan Health Literacy (Schaeffer et al. 2018). In research on accessible communication, we need to focus on these vulnerable groups, especially on people with disabilities, to enable them to participate in health communication on an equal footing with a "maximum of independence" (CRPD paragraph 26 (1)).

In order to be able to access, understand, assess and use health-related information (Sørensen et al. 2012), texts "edited for user-friendliness, as well as a language and text structures easily understood by non-experts" (Schaeffer et al. 2018: 38) are necessary. This emerges from the National Action Plan on Health Literacy (Nationaler Aktionsplan, NAP), which, drawing on Bredel/Maaß (2016), recommends the use of Plain Language as a means of facilitating information seeking and processing for user groups with heterogeneous "reception habits, competence prerequisites and preferences" (Schaeffer et al. 2018: 42f.).

This introductory article combines accessible communication research with health literacy research. It presents intersections between Hildesheim school's accessible communication model (Maaß/Rink 2019) and the integrated model of health literacy (Sørensen et al. 2012) in specialised health texts.

2 Hildesheim school's accessible communication model

Health communication is an area of specialised communication that includes experts and non-experts in the medical field. As such, successful communication is reliant on comprehensibility-enhanced texts that help to bridge the gap between experts and non-experts. To demonstrate the intersections between accessible communication and health literacy research, we need to consider expert-non-expert-communication as our starting position.

Schubert (2007: 210; own translation) defines specialised communication as

> target-oriented, informative, monolingual and multilingual oral and written communication with specialised content carried out by people in the performance of their professional tasks.

Within specialised communication, specialised language is used. Specialised language (Hoffmann 1985: 53, own translation) is defined as

> the totality of all linguistic means that are used in the field of specialised communication in order to ensure understanding between people working in this field.

These two definitions show that health communication plays a special role within specialised communication. Following Weinrich (2015: 393), communicative interactions take place not only among the people who work in the medical field (internal specialised communication, in German: *fachintern*), or among people from various specialities (in German: *interfachlich*), but also with external people (external specialised communication, in German: *fachextern*). One special feature of external specialised communication is the expert-non-expert-communication which is defined as a "systematic asymmetry of knowledge of the communication partners involved" (Bromme/Jucks/Rambow 2004: 176; own translation). One person is the expert who has "disciplinary structured expertise", the other partner is the non-expert who does not have professional experience with regard to the subject in question (ibid). The process of grounding enables understanding between these two communication partners and is defined as follows: Both partners have their own subjective frame of reference consisting of "previous knowledge, attitudes, beliefs and stereotypes as well as [...] dynamic features like currently perceived content, information based on the communication situation and the course of the communication so far" (Bromme/Jucks/Rambow 2004: 179; own translation).

Within a communication setting, these two reference frames meet with the objective "to bring them together to such an extent that their overlap – the so-called common ground – is just sufficient to achieve the respective specific goal of the communication [...]" (ibid.: 178; own translation). Depending on the extent of the knowledge asymmetry, the common ground between the communication partners is either smaller or larger.

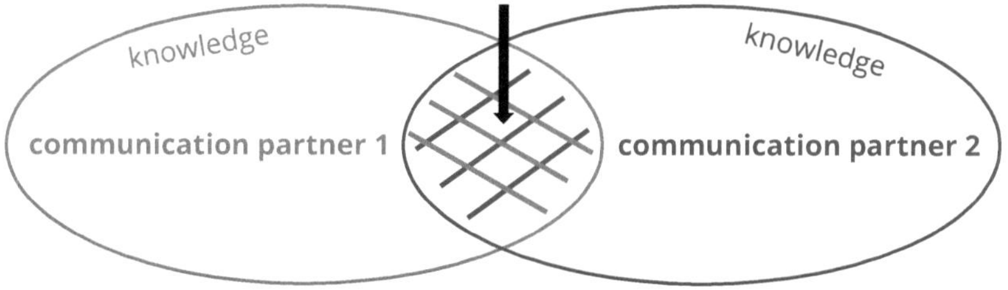

Figure 1: Common ground (Rink 2020: 176; illustration taken from Maaß/Rink (2021))

In the field of specialised communication, there are seven types of constellations that describe the constellation of the communication partners (Kalverkämper 1998: 34f. as in Ahrens 2020: 69):

1. Experts in a field speak about topics of their field of expertise
2. Experts in a field speak about topics of a different field of expertise
3. Experts in different fields speak about topics of one of their fields of expertise
4. Experts in different fields speak about topics of a different field of expertise
5. An expert in a field speaks with a non-expert about topics of their field of expertise
6. An expert in a field speaks with a non-expert about topics of a different field of expertise
7. Non-experts speak about a field of expertise

With regard to the target groups of accessible communication and comprehensibility-enhanced language, Rink (2020: 107; own translation) adds type 5' to this framework:

> The expert in a field speaks with a non-expert who has special communicative needs in terms of accessibility of language because of an impairment. This communication is about subjects from the expert's field and takes place in the manner appropriate to the special needs of the non-expert.

Adequate health communication takes the common ground between sender and recipient into account, also with regards to constellation 5', and the situation in which the text is used (see chapter 3). To explain which further elements need consideration, Hildesheim school's accessible communication model provides a foundation for analysis and research (Figure 2, Hernández Garrido et al. in print, based on Maaß/Rink 2019):

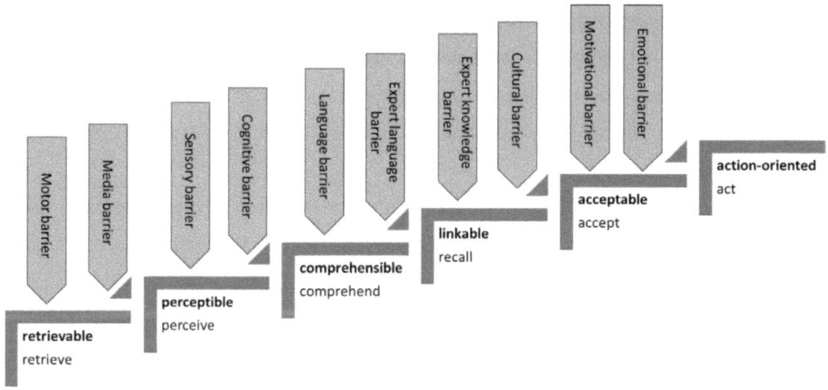

Figure 2: Hildesheim school's accessible communication model with corresponding communication barriers (Hernández Garrido et al. in print, based on Maaß/Rink 2019)

Accessible communication research starts with the assumption that (vulnerable) target groups may be confronted with communication barriers if texts are not adapted to their communicative needs and preferences. This may result in non-participation. The Hildesheim school's accessible communication model is used to identify communication barriers. The model shows the process and the specific features of accessible content that lead to a successful interaction from two perspectives: the user perspective and the text perspective (**bold face**). These two perspectives always belong together: "In order to produce successful products of accessible communication that exhibit the necessary qualities to gain access" we must understand the target groups and their needs as well as the text properties (Maaß 2020: 28).

The model previously mentioned encompasses several steps:

Users must be able to retrieve texts, perceive them using the sensory channels at their disposal, comprehend them, recall them, which is to say texts must link information to the user's previous knowledge, accept them, and be able to use them to take action (Maaß 2020: 27). At the same time, texts must have certain features to enable access to information, e.g., they must be retrievable, perceptible, comprehensible, linkable (to existing knowledge), acceptable and action-enabling (Maaß 2020: 25f.).

For these steps, only a limited working memory capacity is available for the users, even more so for users with a communication impairment (Maaß 2020: 27, Kercher 2013). This capacity may be reduced due to barriers presented by texts. These communication barriers affect different steps within the model.

Retrieval refers to the ability to find information in a communication offer (Lang 2021) while retrievability refers to the corresponding text features. Maaß (2020: 29) points out that "[w]ith regard to the target groups with impairments, retrievability of the information offers is closely related to the groups' media preferences." The ability to retrieve is linked to factors like age, socioeconomic status, group membership and the nature of the disability (ibid. 30). From the text perspective, retrievability "is linked to the mediality of the text offers, to their distribution and location" (ibid), e.g. the media realisation (print, video, radio, etc.), the "path along which the communication offer is delivered to the users" (ibid. 34) and the location on the platform (ibid.).

Retrievability may be hindered by a motor barrier and/or a media barrier. A motor barrier arises when a text's "physical shape is not appropriate for the users" (Maaß 2020: 23), for example using a computer mouse to navigate web pages. A media barrier may arise "if its [the text's] media qualities or means of distribution are not accessible to or used by the target audience" (Maaß 2020: 23). This refers to its realisation (phonic or graphic) as well as the medium used for distribution (ibid).

Perception or perceptibility refers to the abilities and textual features to perceive the information (Maaß 2020: 36). This stage may be obstructed by a sensory barrier and/or a cognitive barrier. A sensory barrier arises if a text is presented in a way that requires a certain sensory channel for successful perception but the recipient cannot use it (Schubert 2016: 17, Rink 2020: 137), e.g. a written text cannot be perceived by a blind person. A cognitive barrier arises if a text is too abstract or complex (Schubert 2016: 18, Rink 2020: 137). A cognitive barrier may arise because the language used or the content structure are too complex (ibid.).

Comprehension or comprehensibility refers to the abilities and features required to comprehend the message of a text and use it to make decisions (Maaß 2020: 41f.). Comprehensibility may be hindered by a language and/or expert language barrier (see Figure 2). A language barrier refers to the language used for the realisation of a text (the code) (Rink 2020: 138). A language barrier emerges when the target group does not understand the language. An expert language barrier emerges when the target group understands the language but not the specific expert language used in a text (Rink 2020: 140), e.g. medical language in health information texts (see also Hill-Madsen 2014, Jensen 2015, Wilkes 2015).

Recall or linking information to existing knowledge refers to the abilities and textual features for linking information in a text to information in the long-term memory (Maaß 2020: 42). This may be hampered by an expert knowledge barrier and/or a cultural barrier. The expert knowledge barrier emerges if expert knowledge is needed to understand the information (Rink 2020: 139), e.g. knowledge about medical processes. The cultural barrier entails for example knowledge of text types and discourse knowledge (Schubert 2016, Rink 2020, Fioravanti/Ahrens forthcoming).

Acceptance or acceptability refers to the degree of agreement that a message may evoke (Lang 2021: 113f. referring to Lucke 1995). Acceptance may be hindered by a motivational and/or an emotional barrier (Lang 2021: 113f.). A motivational barrier may arise due to previous negative experience with reading and/or texts of the same text type (Lang 2021: 119f.) while an emotional barrier may arise due to the situation in which the communication takes place (Lang 2021: 131f.).

The connection between the accessible communication model and the barriers are prototypical: Barriers may arise at different steps during the process depending on the communication situation and the text (Hernández Garrido et al. in print).

3 The integrated model of health literacy and its similarities to the Hildesheim school's accessible communication model

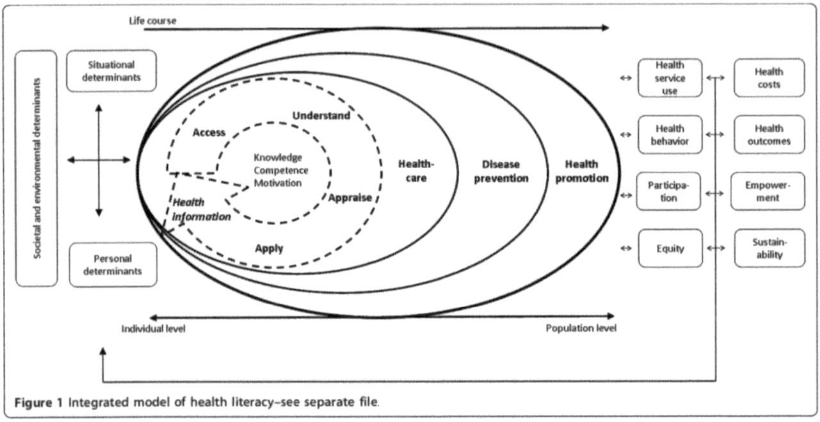

Figure 3: The integrated model of health literacy (Sørensen et al. 2012: 9)

Based on an integrational approach Sørensen et al. (2012: 3) define health literacy as follows:

> Health literacy is linked to literacy and entails people's knowledge, motivation and competences to access, understand, appraise, and apply health information in order to make judgments and take decisions in everyday life concerning healthcare, disease prevention and health promotion to maintain or improve quality of life during the life course. (Sørensen et al. 2012: 3)

Therefore Sørensen et al. (2012: 10) consider the personal, societal and environmental, and the situational determinants of health literacy. They divide health literacy into four main dimensions: access, understand, appraise, and apply. These health literacy dimensions can be found in accessible communication, too (see Chapter 2).

Sørensen et al. (2012: 9, emphasis added) define the health literacy dimensions as follows:

- "Access refers to the ability to **seek**, **find** and **obtain** health information"
- "Understand refers to the ability to **comprehend** the health information that is accessed"
- "Appraise describes the ability to **interpret**, **filter**, **judge** and **evaluate** the health information that has been accessed"
- "Apply refers to the ability to **communicate** and use the information to **make a decision** to maintain and improve health"

These four health literacy dimensions are important in three domains of the health continuum: health care, disease prevention, and health promotion.

	access/obtain information relevant to health	understand information relevant to health	process/appraise information relevant to health	apply/use information relevant to health
health care	ability to access information on medical or clinical issues	ability to understand medical information and derive meaning	ability to interpret and evaluate medical information	ability to make informed decisions on medical issues
disease prevention	ability to access information on risk factors for health	ability to understand information on risk factors and derive meaning	ability to interpret and evaluate information on risk factors for health	ability to make informed decisions on risk factors for health
health promotion	ability to update oneself on determinants of health in the social and physical environment	ability to understand information on determinants of health in the social and physical environment and derive meaning	ability to interpret and evaluate determinants in the social and physical environment	ability to make informed decisions on health determinants in the social and physical environment

Table 1: The four health literacy dimensions applied to the three health domains (adapted from Sørensen et al. 2012: 10)

Table 1 shows what each health literacy dimension means in the context of the respective domain. Sørensen et al. (2012) thus show that the four health literacy dimensions entail slightly different aspects in different settings and that they are flexible to be interpreted according to the function and motive of the health-related information.

Sørensen et al. (2012: 9) define the user aspects of health literacy: literacy, knowledge, motivation, and competences. They further explain that each of the dimension is dependent on "specific cognitive qualities" and "on the quality of the information provided" (Sørensen et al. 2012: 9), and can be used to "[overcome] personal, structural, social and economical barriers to health" (ibid.):

- Access/obtain are determined by "understanding, timing, and trustworthiness"
- Understanding is determined by "expectations, perceived utility, individualization of outcomes and interpretation of causalities"
- Appraisal (and processing) is determined by "the complexity, jargon and partial understandings of the information"
- Effective communication about health information, an element of apply (and use), is determined by comprehension.

Sørensen et al. (2012: 9) thus have similar findings regarding the accessibility of health information as Maaß/Rink (2019, Maaß 2020: 27), and can therefore be compared to the Hildesheim school's accessible communication model (Chapter 2). In the following, the integrated model of health literacy will be assessed from the perspective of accessible communication research[1].

In their health literacy definition (see above), Sørensen et al. (2012: 3) define literacy, knowledge, motivation, and competences as user criteria. They influence and potentially create barriers to the four health literacy dimensions: access, understand, appraise, and apply (see Sørensen et al. 2012: 9). The user criteria can be put into relation to the accessible communication model (see Figure 2): Literacy influences the *language* and *media barrier*. Motivation is

1 Terminology from the field of accessibility research will be printed in italics to improve readability.

represented by the *motivational barrier*. Knowledge influences the common ground between sender and recipient (see above), and therefore plays a role in barriers such as the *expert knowledge barrier* and the *cultural barrier* (see Rink 2020: 139), and at the level of *recall* (see Figure 1).

The four main health literacy dimensions in the model by Sørensen et al. are access, understand, appraise, and apply. These four dimensions are similar to the model of accessible communication proposed by the Hildesheim school, but do not correspond precisely. For one, Sørensen et al. (2012: 9) postulate that "understanding" is part of each of the health literacy dimensions, and thus part of every step within the communication process. The successful interaction through accessible content (see Figure 2) is modelled around the realisation that other elements play a role in accessing information, too (see Maaß 2020: 27). Herein, the process of *comprehension* entails *perception*, *comprehension*, and *recall* (Maaß 2020: 36).

Access, the ability to seek, find, and obtain information (Sørensen et al. 2012: 9), can be placed where *retrievability* and *perceptibility* are in the accessibility model (see Figure 4). As the model by Sørensen et al. is not based around accessibility, sensory channels have not been considered. Therefore, *perceptibility* has not been considered for the integrated model of health literacy.

Trustworthiness, an element that is considered part of *acceptability* in the accessible communication model, is placed at this stage, too (Sørensen et al. 2012: 9). Sørensen et al. hence assume that sources that cannot be trusted are not accessed by health literate users. Under this assumption, *acceptability* would indeed play a large role at the very early stages of accessing a text (cf. Keller in preparation; Lang 2021: 116). However, as a text must be assessed in order to be accepted, the text must first undergo the process of being *retrieved*, *perceived*, *comprehended* and *linked* to previous knowledge. Only then can it be assessed, and as a result of the assessment process *accepted* (Lang 2021: 116). In order to place *acceptability* at the access stage, Sørensen et al. must thus speak of the *acceptance* of an information source, or sender, but not of an individual text (Lang 2021: 117). This places much responsibility with the sending institution: In order to produce texts that will be accessed by the users, the source/sender must be a reputable source that is *accepted* as such by its users.

As previously mentioned, Sørensen et al. (2012) categorise "understand" as an encompassing competence. According to Sørensen et al. (2012: 9) user expectations and perceived utility for the user facilitate understanding. This is confirmed by *comprehensibility* and *accessibility research* (Kercher 2013, Schubert 2016, Rink 2020): Expectations of text types and text topics guide the user's expectations on a text (Brinker et al. 2014: 139). Perceived utility enhances the *motivation* to read a text (Lang 2021: 123f.) and can thus help *comprehension*. Sørensen et al. (2012: 9) name the individualisation and the interpretation of causalities as further prerequisites for understanding. However, these two factors must be seen rather as outcomes of good *comprehension*. Both are processes of connecting the information within the text to prior knowledge and thus, from the viewpoint of the Hildesheim school's accessible communication model, fall under *linkable*.

Furthermore, Sørensen et al. name the elements complexity and jargon at the appraisal stage when they are elements of *comprehension* (see Figure 1). Expert language entails complex constructions that take up working memory capacity, thus impeding text *comprehension* (for working memory see Kercher 2013: 79f.). Appraisal is defined as the ability to interpret, filter, judge, and evaluate (Sørensen et al. 2012: 9) and is thus dependent on *comprehension*. *Expert language* elements like complexity and jargon thus impede appraisal only indirectly: It impedes comprehension, and poor comprehension does not allow for proper appraisal.

The abilities of appraisal "interpret" and "filter" (see above) should be both elements of *comprehension* and of appraisal: In the comprehension process, interpretation is relevant on the levels of segments, sentences and the text (Kercher 2013: 74), and filtering is important on the text level, to alleviate the burden on the working memory. Important information is kept in the working memory while less important information is left aside, thus filtered (Kercher 2013: 74.). The important information is later interpreted on the text level to create a complete picture of the text (Kercher 2013: 78). After *comprehension*, the information is again interpreted and filtered, taking into account situational factors like source/sender and prior knowledge to discern relevant and correct information (Kercher 2013: 70), making "interpret" and "filter" also elements of appraisal. The two terms are thus ill-defined by Sørensen et al. and can be interpreted to fit comprehension and appraisal alike. The lines between understanding and appraisal in Sørensen et al.'s model are thus blurred. The appraisal of a text, if well defined, can be placed at the levels of *linkability* and *acceptability* in accessible communication (see Figure 4).

Sørensen et al.'s health literacy dimension "apply (and use)" focuses solely on the aspects of communicating, judging information, and making decisions. It does not consider actual action that is taken or not taken after the text reception process. Considering the model's background in medicine and public health (Sørensen et al. 2012: 9), actual (health) behaviour can hardly be part of it, as is evident, for example, in the fact that knowledge of smoking risks does not automatically lead to cessation (see e.g. Eklund et al. 2012). The model of accessible communication, however, is not health-information specific and cannot make a distinction between making decisions and actual action. Here, being enabled to make a decision and actual action are both elements of "act".

The convergence between the two models is visualised in Figure 4:

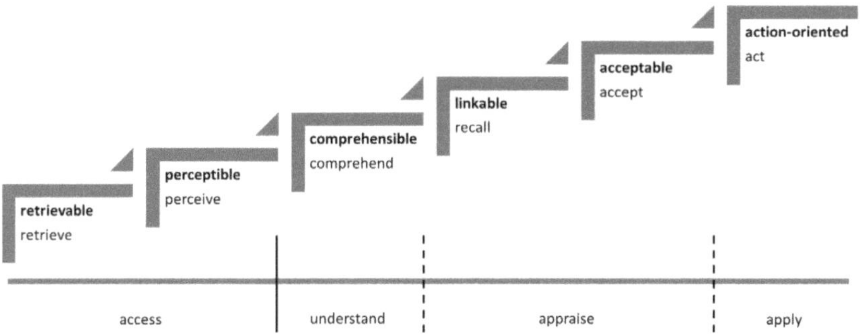

Figure 4: The four health literacy dimensions applied to the model of accessible communication

As explained above (Table 1), the four main health literacy dimensions can be applied to three public health dimensions: health care, disease prevention, and health promotion. These three aspects frame the communication situation in which a text is situated. The four main health literacy dimensions are defined differently according to the dimension, which is to say according to the *communication situation*. As different user scenarios have been taken into account, the integrated model of health literacy can be adapted to specific text types and their communication situations. It is similar to Hildesheim school's accessible communication model, showing converging results from two different research fields and traditions. From the point of view of accessible communication, Sørensen et al.'s flexible and interpretable model can be re-organised to fit field-specific requirements.

4 On the Handbook *Accessibility – Health Literacy – Health Information. Interdisciplinary Approaches to an Emerging Field of Communication*

This handbook aims to show direct links between research and practice in accessible communication, health information and health literacy. Nine contributions shed light onto those connections from a *methodical, text*, and *user perspective*. The authors come from different fields with diverse research traditions, but they all see the relevance of interdisciplinary approaches in an emerging field of action that focuses on communicating accessible health related information and methods to specific target groups:

Dalemans et al. discuss how accessible questionnaires can be helpful for vulnerable groups when they take part in Patient-Reported Outcome Measures (PROMs). They present a Communication Friendly Measurement Guideline, a tool that supports the creation of questionnaires that are communication friendly.

Häberle shows how good organisational health literacy, i.e. the effective incorporation of health literacy into organisational action, improves accessibility. She addresses access to as well as communication and navigation within organisations, illuminating accessibility from the point of health organisations.

Hörner describes how the implementation of Plain Language texts on the website of the leading health publisher in Germany (Wort & Bild Verlag) was achieved and which difficulties have been faced.

Keller focusses on elderly users and their media access, preferences, and competences to discuss key factors for retrievability and acceptability of digital health information in this target group.

Kröger and Ahrens describe a method to analyse health information texts for intralingual translation. They present methods used in their research projects to determine potential barriers in health texts.

Leyerer et al. report on experiences of the German Cancer Research Centre on translating evidence-based health information in Easy Language and Plain Language.

Michele and Silke discuss action-orientation in teaching-learning concepts for health staff. The authors detail health literacy of health professionals and their competence in transferring health literacy onto their patients, and connect these two aspects to the concept of vocational action competence.

Pedrini analyses the use of passive voice and related structures in layperson summaries of clinical trials. She designed a corpus of layperson summaries in English and German and the corresponding English texts for medical experts and checks both frequency and qualitative aspects of passive diathesis.

Rink and Schulz explain how data collection methods need to be adapted to allow for research with people with cognitive impairments. They discuss linguistic, conceptual and medial strategies to improve data collections and obtain valid results.

Literature

Ahrens, Sarah (2020): "Easy Language and Administrative Texts: Second Language Learners as a Target Group". In: Hansen-Schirra, Silvia/Maaß, Christiane (eds.): *Easy Language Research: Text and User Perspectives*. Berlin: Frank & Timme. Easy – Plain – Accessible Vol. 2, pp. 67–97.

Bredel, Ursula/Maaß, Christiane (2016): *Leichte Sprache. Theoretische Grundlagen, Orientierung für die Praxis*. Berlin: Duden.

Brinker, Klaus/Cölfen, Hermann/Pappert, Steffen (2014): *Linguistische Textanalyse: Eine Einführung in Grundbegriffe und Methoden* (8. Aufl.). Berlin: Erich Schmidt Verlag.

Bromme, Rainer/Jucks, Regina/Rambow, Riklef (2004): "Experten-Laien-Kommunikation im Wissensmanagement". In: Reinmann, Gabi/Mandl,

Heinz (eds.): *Der Mensch im Wissensmanagement: Psychologische Konzepte zum besseren Verständnis und Umgang mit Wissen.* Göttingen: Hogrefe, pp. 176–188.

CRPD. Convention on the Rights of Persons with Disabilities. <https://www.un.org/development/desa/disabilities/convention-on-the-rights-of-persons-with-disabilities.html>

Eklund, Britt-Marie/Nilsson, Siv/Hedman, Linnea/Lindberg, Inger (2012): "Why do smokers diagnosed with COPD not quit smoking? – a qualitative study". In: *Tobacco Induced Diseases* 10 (17).

Fioravanti, Chiara/Ahrens, Sarah (forthcoming): "Cultural implications in Easy Language texts for migrants: theoretical considerations and insights from practice in Germany and in Italy". In: Deilen, Silvana/Hansen-Schirra, Silvia/Hernández Garrido, Sergio/Maaß, Christiane/Tardel, Anke (eds.): *Easy Language and Accessible Communication.*

Hernández Garrido, Sergio/Maaß, Christiane/Becker, Lidia/Pedraza, Maria Betulia (in print): "Multimodal health communication towards vulnerable groups in Colombia in the context of the COVID-19 crisis". In: Schmidt, Franziska/Jaki, Sylvia/Mandl, Thomas (eds.): *Wissen um Corona. Wissenschaftskommunikation, Informationsverhalten, Diskurs.* Hildesheim: Universitätsverlag.

Hill-Madsen, Aage (2014): *Derivation and transformation: Strategies in lay-oriented intralingual translation.* Aarhus University: Department of Business Communication.

Hoffmann, Lothar (1985): *Kommunikationsmittel Fachsprache. Eine Einführung.* 2. neu bearb. Auflage Tübingen: Narr.

Jensen, Matilde Nisbeth (2015): "Optimising comprehensibility in interlingual translation: The need for intralingual translation". In: Maksymski, Karin/Gutermuth, Silke/Hansen-Schirra, Silvia (eds.): *Translation and Comprehensibility.* TransÜD Vol. 72. Berlin: Frank & Timme, pp. 163–194.

Kalverkämper, Hartwig (1998): "Rahmenbedingungen für die Fachkommunikation". In: Hoffmann, Lothar/Kalverkämper, Hartwig/Wiegand, Herbert E. (eds.): *Fachsprachen. Ein internationales Handbuch zur Fachsprachenforschung und Terminologiewissenschaft. 1. Halbband.* Berlin, New York: De Gruyter, pp. 24–43.

Keller, Loraine (in prep.): *Verständlichkeitsoptimierte Medizinkommunikation. Akzeptabilität und Akzeptanz von Texten in Einfacher und Leichter Sprache.* Manuscript of dissertation. Hildesheim: Universität Hildesheim.

Kercher, Jan (2013): *Verstehen und Verständlichkeit von Politikersprache. Verbale Bedeutungsvermittlung zwischen Politikern und Bürgern.* Wiesbaden: Springer.

Lang, Katrin (2021): *Auffindbarkeit, Wahrnehmbarkeit, Akzeptabilität. Webseiten von Behörden in Leichter Sprache vor dem Hintergrund der rechtlichen Lage.* Berlin: Frank & Timme. Easy – Plain – Accessible Vol. 10.

Lucke, Doris (1995): *Akzeptanz: Legitimität in der "Abstimmungsgesellschaft".* Opladen: Leske + Budrich.

Maaß, Christiane/Rink, Isabel (2019): "Über das Handbuch Barrierefreie Kommunikation". In: Maaß, Christiane/Rink, Isabel (eds.): *Handbuch Barrierefreie Kommunikation.* Kommunikation – Partizipation – Inklusion Vol. 3. Berlin: Frank & Timme, pp. 17–25.

Maaß, Christiane/Rink, Isabel (2021): Translating Legal Texts into Easy Language. In: *Journal of Open Access to Law* 9 (1).

Maaß, Christiane (2020): *Easy Language – Plain Language – Easy Language Plus. Balancing Comprehensibility and Acceptability.* Berlin: Frank & Timme. Easy – Plain – Accessible Vol. 3.

Rink, Isabel (2020): *Rechtskommunikation und Barrierefreiheit. Zur Übersetzung juristischer Informations- und Interaktionstexte in Leichte Sprache.* Berlin: Frank & Timme. Easy – Plain – Accessible Vol. 1.

Schaeffer, Doris/Vogt, Dominique/Berens, Eva-Maria/Hurrelmann, Klaus (2016): *Gesundheitskompetenz der Bevölkerung in Deutschland – Ergebnisbericht.* Bielefeld: Universität Bielefeld. DOI: 10.2390/0070-pub-29088450.

Schaeffer, Doris/Hurrelmann, Klaus/Bauer, Ulrich/Kolpatzik, Kai (2018.): *National Action Plan Health Literacy. Promoting Health Literacy in Germany.* Berlin: KomPart.

Schaeffer, Doris/Berens, Eva-Maria/Gille, Svea/Griese, Lennert/Klinger, Julia/de Sombre, Steffen/Vogt, Dominique/Hurrelmann, Klaus (2021): *Gesundheitskompetenz der Bevölkerung in Deutschland – vor und während der Corona Pandemie: Ergebnisse des HLS-GER 2. Bielefeld: Interdisziplinäres Zentrum für Gesundheitskompetenz-forschung (IZGK)*, Universität Bielefeld. DOI: <https://doi.org/10.4119/unibi/2950305>

et al. 2016). The language is complex and uses unfamiliar (medical) vocabulary. In addition, the questionnaires are often too long and overloaded with information on one page. For people who are communication vulnerable, these PROMs are often very challenging (de Boer et al. 2013, Stans 2013) (for an explanation of communication vulnerability, see Figure 1).

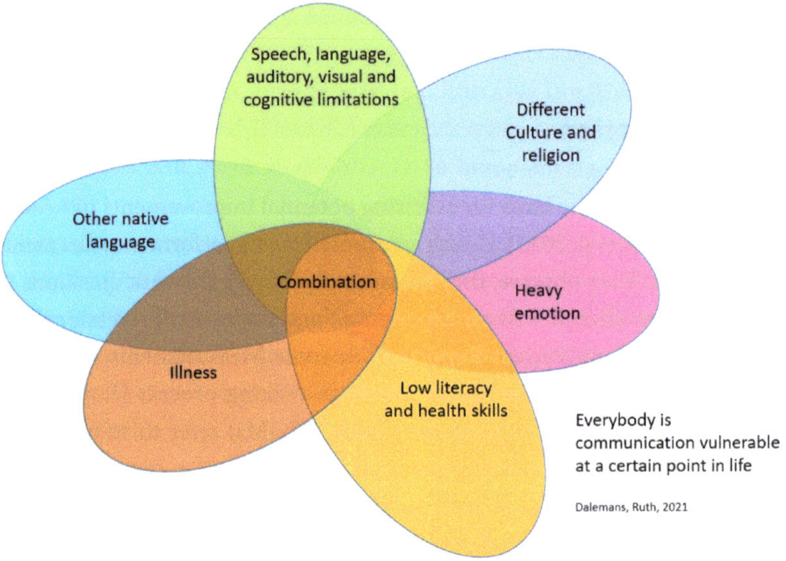

Figure 1: Communication vulberability: people experience difficulties in understanding and expressing information in certain social contexts due to certain condition(s)

They sometimes just tick an answer without really understanding the question, or it takes professionals a long time to clarify the question. As a result, clients cannot properly share their needs, wishes for treatment and experiences with their care. The questionnaires then do not measure what they are supposed to measure; the measurements are not valid. As a result, care professionals are not able to match the care to clients' real problems (for an overview on how to adapt data collection methods to specific target groups' communicative needs, see Rink/Schulz in this volume).

When clients are confronted with an incomprehensible questionnaire, they lose their trust in the relationship with the professional, get frustrated, and lose their energy (Dalemans 2018, see also Keller in this volume). Professionals on the other hand, have a feeling of wasting time and do not trust the received data. Therefore, it is important that questionnaires are designed to be communication-friendly. Questionnaires are communication-friendly if they measure reliably and validly because they are adapted to the communicative abilities of the client and enable the client to understand the questions and answer them adequately without much effort or time (Dalemans 2018).

The majority of questionnaires, however, are written at a higher level of language complexity than is likely to be understood by the persons intended to complete them. This is of significance, given that researchers and practitioners alike rely on data from PROMs in drawing conclusions (Taylor et al. 2019). For the large group of clients with communication challenges and their professionals, it is therefore important to investigate how questionnaires can be made more communication-friendly (Dalemans et al. 2009).

We therefore examined which requirements should be met in questionnaires and how they should be designed for people who are communication vulnerable, so that care professionals can obtain valid and reliable information to organize the care process in the best possible way together with their clients.

2 Method used in the project 'See and hear the client'

2.1 Design

We answered the central research question – which requirements should be met in questionnaires and how they should be designed for people who are communication vulnerable, so that care professionals can obtain valid and reliable information to organize the care process in the best possible way together with their clients? – by means of design-based research in three work packages (see Table 1). This design entails researchers and relevant stakeholders collaborating in an iterative process in which data collection (qualitative and quantitative) and the insights gained are continuously used to inform subsequent design phases (Barab 2004, Collins 2004). Relevant stakeholders in this project were: adults who are communication vulnerable due to an Acquired

Brain Injury (ABI), care professionals working with these people, experts (in data visualization, communication, language), client representatives, researchers, lecturers and students. They all worked together in the project group, the steering group and/or within several co-design meetings.

Work package 1	Exploring current use and experiences with existing questionnaires with 30 participants: 15 people who are communication vulnerable due to an ABI and their professionals.
Work package 2	Developing a set of redesign rules Redesigning three existing questionnaires
Work package 3	Testing the clinimetric properties (comprehensibility, feasibility, test-retest reliability and content validity) of the communication-friendly versions of these three questionnaires in 177 people who are communication vulnerable due to an ABI.

Table 1: Goals of each work package

This contribution will focus on work packages 1 and 2 and the comprehensibility of the three redesigned questionnaires.

2.2 Setting, recruitment and population

The research took part at three different care facilities: 1) a care organization in the South of the Netherlands providing supported living and living arrangements to people with severe acquired, intellectual and developmental disabilities; 2) a care organization in the South of the Netherlands providing care (living arrangements, nursing care and wellbeing) to elderly clients and clients with a chronic condition; 3) a rehabilitation centre in the North of the Netherlands providing rehabilitation services to adults and children. In addition, participants were recruited in some local aphasia centres. Care professionals and clients were recruited via the contact persons of these facilities. Care professionals had to work with clients with neurogenic communication disorders on a weekly basis and had to be authorized to use the questionnaire(s). Clients had to be communication vulnerable due to aphasia, dysarthria, cognitive communication disorder and/or a verbal apraxia. Clients were excluded if they suffered from dementia phase 3 or psychiatric disorders.

2.3 Intervention: three questionnaires

The three existing questionnaires to be adjusted in this project were:

- Aphasia Impact Questionnaire-NL (Dutch version: AIQ-NL): Investigates the impact of aphasia on communication, participation and wellbeing (Swinburn 2018; Wielaert et al. 2018). It contains 21 items using 1 scale.
- Computer Assisted Form of the Adjusted Dutch version of the Swallow Quality of life Questionnaire (CAF-aDSWALQOL): Investigates the impact of swallowing problems on quality of life (Simpelaere et al. 2017): It contains 50 items divided into 5 subscales Feelings (11 items), Body Complaints and Symptoms (15 items), Daily meal (7 items), Daily life (6 items), and General Questions (11 items).
- Client satisfaction questionnaire Stichting Gehandicaptenzorg Limburg (CSQ – SGL): Investigates clients' satisfaction with the day care facilities of SGL (self-developed unpublished questionnaire). It contains 31 items grouped into the following subscales: (1) Daily activities (contains 6 items), (2) Employees and volunteers (8 items), (3) Information (3 items), (4) SGL Health care plan (4 items), (5) Safety (4 items), and Building and feeding (3 items).

We chose three totally different questionnaires with regard to aim, target group and layout in order to gather different and rich experiences and to enlarge the generalizability of the design requirements. In each setting, the same target group is addressed, namely people who are communication vulnerable due to an ABI, however the focus in each setting is a little different. In the setting of the DSWAL-QOL, people need to have swallowing problems in addition to the neurogenic communication disorders, whereas this does not need to be the case in the other settings. In the setting of the AIQ-NL, the people need to have at least aphasia because of the measured impact of aphasia in the AIQ-NL. The original

AIQ-NL and CSQ – SGL are presented in their paper version. The DSWAL-QOL had already been digitalized in a previous study (Jans/Sondeijker 2018).

2.4 Data collection and -analysis

Work package 1: Current use and experiences with existing questionnaires

	Clients		Age range	Etiology
	woman	man		
AIQ-NL	n=2	n=3	48–64 year	Stroke
DSWAL-QOL	n=3	n=2	52–83 year	Stroke, ALS
CTO SGL	n=2	n=3	58–77 year	Stroke, Vascular dementia

We conducted observations of the current use of the three questionnaires (n=15, 5 from each participating care facility) focusing on: clients' reactions to visualizations and display of language, meaning of language and interaction between clients and professionals. After the observations, clients and professionals were interviewed based on the researchers' observations, focusing on critical factors with regard to comprehensibility and on contextual factors and conditions, as well as on the digital competence with regard to the DSWAL-Qol. Observations and interviews were audiotaped and transcribed verbatim. Deductive content analysis using the categories visualization, display of language and meaning of language (semantic and grammatical structure) as a framework was applied (Elo 2008).

Work package 2: Redesigning the three questionnaires

We organized co-creation and brainstorm sessions with stakeholders, in which different strategies and alternative solutions were formulated in combination with evidence-based strategies. Ultimately, a decision was made by the project team for high potential strategies. Based on that, 20 different prototypes were developed by Metrisquare, a Dutch company specialized in developing and adjusting measurement instruments for care, especially focusing on visual presentation. The prototypes consisted of simple statements with a dichotomous answering scale in which one or more strategies were applied (visualization, representation, i.e. layout, and meaning of language, i.e. linguistic structures). We then pilot tested the prototypes using a cross-over design with 20 participants who were communication vulnerable. Eye-tracking (Tobii Eyetracking) in combination with the think-aloud method (Charters 2003) were used to collect data about which strategies worked the best. Using a Tobii Eyetracking device, eye movements were monitored for each prototype, providing insights into the cognitive processes involved while answering the questions. Outcome measures were: order and lengths of visual fixation, the time between looking at the question and giving the answer and the correctness of answers. During the testing via eye-tracking, a think aloud interview technique was used to stimulate the participant to immediately share his or her thoughts about the prototype with the researcher. Interviews were transcribed and analysed using inductive content analysis (Elo 2008). The quantitative data gathered though eye-tracking was described in an Excel file with regard to duration of fixations and order of Eyetracking in relation to the response time and number of correct responses per prototype; both individual and group results were analysed.

Based on the results of the pilot-testing a set of redesign rules was decided upon by the project team, and the three questionnaires were adjusted accordingly. The redesign rules were processed into a generic Communication-friendly Measurement Guideline.

Work package 3: Comprehensibility and clinimetric properties

Phase 3 consisted of a comprehensibility study and a study testing clinimetric properties (content validity and test-retest reliability) in 177 people who are communication vulnerable due to an ABI of the communication-friendly versions of the three questionnaires. This chapter focuses on the comprehensibility study. The methods and results of the clinimetric properties will be published soon.

The comprehensibility study aimed to measure whether clients perceive the adjusted versions of the questionnaires as more comprehensible than the original version. Data collection took place through structured observations of the administration of a number of items from the original version of the three questionnaires (five items per questionnaires that were found to be difficult in work package 1), versus the redesigned version of the three questionnaires in combination with interviews with end-users (see Figure 2), thus each participant completed 15 original and 15 new questions. Twenty end-users (12 men and eight women) participated. Half of them (n=10) had suffered a stroke, six of them were diagnosed with aphasia, four with Parkinson's disease. Other Acquired Brain Injuries (ABI) with both cognitive and language processing problems were known in three persons. The cause of the ABI was not reported for three persons. The mean age was 66.4 (sd=14.9; range 35–88 years). Most people (n=13) completed the questionnaire independently. In the case of seven people (mainly the elderly), the test leader clicked n the answers.

Figure 2 shows an example of an original item versus an adapted item from the AIQ-NL. In the modified item we used a colour photograph, shortened the question, adapted the answer option to the question, added a navigation bar so that the person could see how many items were still to come, changed the font size and font type based upon the Communication-friendly Measurement Guideline (Dalemans et al. 2022).

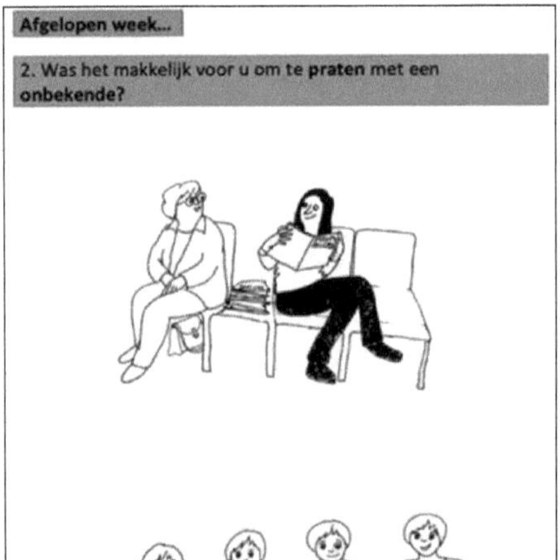

Figure 2A: Original item version AIQ-NL

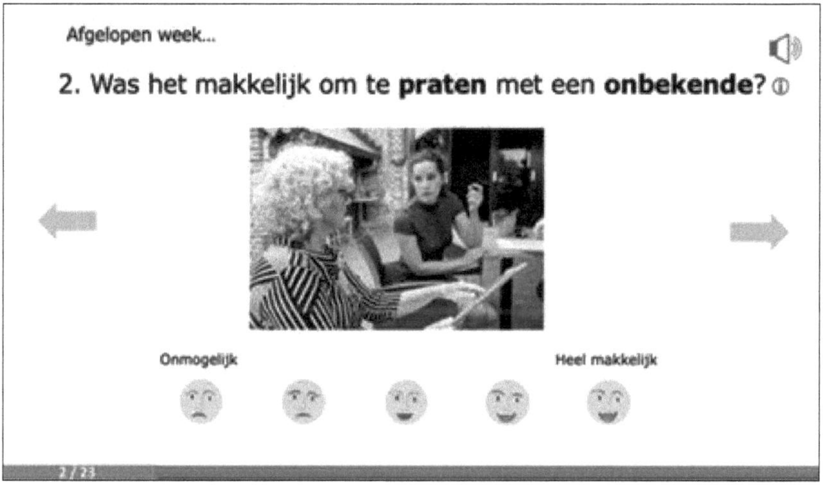

Figure 2B: Communication-friendly version E-AIQ-NL used in the comprehensibility study

Observations focused on: degree of independence, and number of questions asked. The participant filled in the questions. In addition, the researcher asked a number of open questions to the participant (see Appendix 2) to gain insight into the client's opinion. Observations and interviews were audiotaped and transcribed and analysed using inductive content analysis (Elo 2008).

2.5 Collecting data with communication vulnerable people

Collecting data with people who are communication vulnerable requires using communication supportive tools and strategies (see Rink/Schulz in this volume). We used several communication supportive tools and strategies tailored to the individual needs and capacities of the participants, such as: creating a low-stimulus environment, using pencil and paper, non-verbal gestures, photos and support using the digital context if necessary, for example clicking the mouse when the person asked for it. The interviewer always adjusted her communicative style to the participant (short sentence, highly frequent words, low speed of speech, visualizing key concepts, sufficient pauses). Furthermore, interviewers encouraged the participant to honestly say when he/she is tired. Next to using these tools and strategies during the interviews, all written communication (e.g. information letters and informed consent) were made communication-friendly (using the results of the project immediately) (Stans et al. 2017).

2.6 Trustworthiness

We applied several strategies to ensure the trustworthiness of the project. We used member check to safeguard that results were an actual representation of participants' experiences. For clients, we made communication-friendly summaries of the interviews/observations. Furthermore, we applied peer review as we regular held reflective data sessions with the whole project team. Moreover, to gather data we used several different methods (interviews, observations, eye tracking) (Lincoln/Guba 1985).

Ethical considerations

The study was approved by the Medical Ethics Committee of Zuyderland – Zuyd METCZ20190050.

3 Results

3.1 Work package 1: Current experiences with existing questionnaires

Based upon the interviews and observations seven main themes arose: formulation of questions, response options, layout, length, navigation, clients' characteristics, support needed.

Theme	Results
Formulation of questions	Participants had difficulties understanding specific words, and more abstract concepts such as 'isolation'. The questions comprised difficult words and the formulation of the sentences was often too complex. In some cases, one question actually contained two questions.
Response options	Participants experienced difficulties with questionnaires in which the response options greatly varied. If there were only two answer options (Yes/No), participants would have liked a 'not applicable' – option. The CSQ – SGL contained no visual support for the response options. The AIQ contained drawings which the participants found helpful, however participants experienced these as too negative. The DSWAL-QOL used different answer scales per question, which was experienced as complex.
Layout	The CSQ – SGL questionnaire's font was too small and the questionnaire contained too many questions on one page. No visual support was available. The AIQ contained drawings, however some of the drawings were experienced as confusing, for example a drawing of someone dropping a vase to support the word shame. The DSWAL-QOL used sclera pictograms to support the question, those were sometimes too abstract.
Length	The length of the CSQ – SGL questionnaire was found to be too long, the length of the AIQ questionnaire was evaluated as good. The DSWAL-QOL was found to be long, but acceptable.
Navigation	Navigation was experienced as difficult in two questionnaires (CSQ – SGL, AIQ). Participants needed support from a professional. In the SGL questionnaire this was mainly due to the complex layout and many questions on one page. The AIQ is interview-based and the professional often indicated how many questions were left before reaching the end of the questionnaire. In the DSWAL-QOL a navigation tool was already used. Participants did not mention this tool as helpful, nor as disturbing.
Wish for independent use	Clients expressed the desire to fill in the questionnaires more independently. A professional can be present, but they would like to answer the questions as independently as possible.
Support needed	The professionals gave extensive support in the use of the questionnaires: reading questions out loud, giving examples, pointing to questions, checking answers, navigating and giving visual information for the answering scale.

Table 2: Main themes in the experiences with existing questionnaires

- The target group of the guideline is everyone who professionally uses questionnaires in contact with people who are vulnerable in communication. These are paramedics, medics, nurses, psychologists, social workers, municipal officials.
- The guide can be used in three ways: 1) in the development of a new questionnaire where the whole guide can be used as a guide, 2) in the communication-friendly adaptation of a self-created questionnaire, where, depending on the time available, one can choose to adapt one aspect first (e.g. display of language) or to adapt several aspects at the same time, 3) in the communication-friendly adaptation of an existing validated questionnaire: this first requires contact with the original author of the questionnaire.
- The guide should be easy to use, with unambiguous instructions. This also means that it should be concise, attractive and easy to understand.
- Applying the guide should lead to an overview of action points with which the professional can immediately set to work to make the questionnaire communication-friendly.

The project group developed the guideline in several sessions, each feedback round leading to further adjustments whereby the above-mentioned criteria were always compared to the draft guideline. Subsequently, the project group joined forces with a graphic designer to make the guide attractive and manageable by designing an interactive PDF file. This guideline aims to support professionals in evaluating how communication-friendly a questionnaire is, and provides guidance on how they can (easily) adjust/improve the questionnaire. The guideline is divided into five themes: visualization (n=11), display of language (n=10), meaning of language (i.e. semantic and grammatical structure) (n=11), response scale (n=3), and structure (n=5). It contains a total of 39 subsequent items that professionals can use for the evaluation and adjustment of questionnaires. The guide starts with a short introduction on the importance of communication-friendly measurement and a description of some of the advantages of applying it. This is followed by a scientific explanation of how the guide came into being. Then the professional is instructed on the use of the guide and the steps to follow. Subsequently, the professional can really get to work. In an overview, the professional can check which part he or she wants to start with first (see Figure 3).

Visualization	Display of language	Meaning of language	Response scale	Structure
Picture in colour	Use of white space	Priming concepts	Structure text and image	Use of a grid
GIF	1 item per page	Word length	Colour of answer	Option for backward
Image activity	1 sentence per line	Language level	Answering options	Option for proceeding
Image object	Readability font	High frequent words		Option for pausing
Image emotion	Font size	Highly imaginable words		Audio support for text
Context of image	Bold font keywords	Avoid negation		
Identification	Line spacing 1.5	Active sentences		
Limit details	Text image	Avoid derivatives		
Use of metaphors	Text GIF	Sentence length (8–12 words)		
Contrast	Display of numbers	Priming: structure of information		
		Consistency		

Figure 3: Overview redesign rules

The guideline is presented in a 'smart PDF' format in which professionals can tick boxes for which item has to be adjusted to make the questionnaire communication-friendly. In addition, for each item a 'traffic light system' is used:

the item is red (needs adjustment), yellow (improvements can be made), green (no actions needed). At the end, the user receives an overview of the actions needed to make the questionnaire communication-friendly.

Using the Communication-Friendly Measurement Guideline

Anyone who uses and/or develops questionnaires can benefit from applying the guideline. Any adjustment that leads to better use of the questionnaire by people who are vulnerable to communication is valuable:

- When developing a new questionnaire: use the Communication-Friendly Measurement Guideline from the start.
- When adapting an existing questionnaire: by using the checklist in the guideline, it immediately becomes clear how communication-friendly the questionnaire already is and which steps can be taken to make it even more communication-friendly, for example by adding visualizations and formulating the questions simply, actively, positively and briefly.
- When adapting a validated questionnaire: some parts are easy to adjust, such as font and line spacing. However, to adjust wording or add visualizations, the developer of the questionnaire should be contacted, or contact the researchers of the project “See & Hear the Client”. Together, we can examine how questionnaires can be adapted in a communication-friendly way without influencing their validity. After all, everyone is entitled to communication-friendly measurements.

The guideline can also be used to design other types of written communication in a communication-friendly way.

3.3 Work package 3: Testing the comprehensibility of the communication-friendly version of these three questionnaires

The communication-friendly version (CF version) of the items of the three questionnaires were experienced as easier and more understandable by the participants in comparison to the original items. It was indicated that this new version was the more understandable due to better visibility (possibility to adjust the background colour according to preference) and use of colour pictures.

Furthermore, they found the read-aloud function helpful to comprehend the question as well as the visual support of the answer scale. They judged the connection of the answer scale to the question as good. For a small number of participants, the paper version is preferred because of its tangibility and the possibility to write on it. This supports the cognitive processing process. Paper and e-versions should therefore exist side by side. As many aspects as possible from the Communication-friendly Measurement Guideline should be applied in the questionnaire.

Choosing the background colour

In total, 80 % of the participants say that they like choosing a background colour because they have problems with their vision. This shows that the CF-version is preferred over the original. Two participants (13 %) do not find it necessary to choose a background colour because they have no problems with their vision and another participant says it does not matter. One participant (7 %) could not answer the question because of severe comprehension problems.

Better understanding

The majority of the participants indicated that the CF-version ensures better comprehension due to high frequency words and short sentences; 86 % indicated that choosing a background colour as well as the use of short sentences and high frequency words helps to understand the question better because they can see and read it better. One participant (7 %) could not answer the question because of severe comprehension problems. The remaining participant (7 %) indicated that background colour did not contribute to the comprehensibility of the question because they did not experience any problems with their vision.

Listening to the question again

Of the participants, 67 % indicated that re-listening helped them understand the question better because they could not read properly and that the CF-version was therefore more comprehensible and came out best. A small number of the participants (20 %) indicated that it did not contribute to the understanding of the questions because reading went well. The remaining two participants (13 %) could not answer this question because of comprehension problems.

Clarity of visual support

Colour pictures are perceived to be the clearest: There were 3 participants (27 %) who found the black and white line drawing the clearest as they found it easier to look at. Three participants (20 %) found both the black and white line drawing and the colour photos clear. One participant (7 %) could not answer this question due to comprehension problems. The other participants (53 %) found the colour pictures the most clear as they showed real people and they could identify with the situation. All found visual support to be an added value compared to the absence of visual support.

Difficulty of answering scale

In general, the response scale of the CF-version appeared to be the easiest to fill in, which is why this version came out on top: 20 % found the paper response scales the easiest to fill in because they found the little figures easier and because they could tick them on paper. A total of 60 % found the answer keys on the laptop easier to fill in because of the clear and distinctive colour of the faces and the logical answer options. One participant (7 %) found them both equally easy and the remaining two participants (13 %) could not answer this question due to comprehension problems.

Comprehensibility of original version versus CF-version

The CF-version was found to be the most understandable by 46 % of the participants because it was more visible and because the questions were presented textually, visually and orally. Only 27 % of the participants found the paper version the most comprehensible because it was tangible and they could write on it. The remaining four participants (27 %) found both versions equally understandable.

Level of difficulty original version versus CF-version

The CF-version was perceived to be the easiest; 46 % indicated that they found the CF-version the easiest because the question was presented orally, because it was easier to read because of the background colour and because they did not have to write, but could just point/click. The participants who did not experience this (40 %) found the original version easier because it was more tangible. One participant found both questionnaires equally easy (7 %). One participant (7 %) could not answer this question because of comprehension problems.

More autonomy

The CF-version gave more autonomy to the participants. Participants were in control of the pace of the CF-version, could make their own choices and could decide whether they wanted to hear a question again. This gave them a feeling of more independence:

> "Even though it's hard to control a laptop myself, I do feel more independent."

4 Conclusion

In this project, a collaborative effort between researchers, clients and experts has been made to develop a 'Communication-Friendly Measurement Guideline' using the method of design-oriented research. By involving experts on language and visualization, professionals and especially the key-users from the start of the project systematically and testing the adjustments, the results fit the purpose. Strategies to make questionnaires communication-friendly have been described in five domains (visualizations, representation of language, meaning of language, answer scale and structure). Every strategy that is applied is a step closer to a communication-friendly questionnaire. This research project has shown that questionnaires are often not communication-friendly. A Communication-friendly Measurement Guideline has been developed in collaboration with key-users and other stakeholders. The application of the guideline in ad-

Clerehan, R./Guillemin, F./Epstein, J./Buchbinder, R. (2016): "Using the Evaluative Linguistic Framework for Questionnaires to Assess Comprehensibility of Self-Reprot Health Questionnaires". In: *Value in Health*, 19 (4), pp. 335–342.

Collins, A./Joseph, D./Bielaczyc, K. (2004): "Design Research: Theoretical and Methodological Issues". In: *Journal of the Learning Sciences*, 3, pp. 15–42.

Dalemans, Ruth; Stans, Steffy; von Helden-Lenzen, Stephanie; Lemmens, Jessie; Ummels, Darcy; Cornips, Stephanie; et al. (2021): *Leidraad Communicatievriendelijk meten. Zuyd University of Applied Sciences. Report.* https://doi.org/10.25385/zuyd.16782985.v1

Dalemans, R. (2018a): *Anders Meten met beelden: communicatievriendelijk meten*. Heerlen: LIME, Zuyd.

Dalemans, R. (2018b): *Zie en Hoor de client: herontwerpen van vragenlijsten voor mensen met een Niet Aangeboren Hersenletsel*. Stichting Innovatie Alliantie.

Dalemans, R./Wade, D. T./van den Heuvel, W. J./de Witte, L. (2009): "Facilitating the participation of people with aphasia in research: a description of strategies". In: *Clinical Rehabilitation*, 23 (10), pp. 948–959.

de Boer, D./Delnoij, D./Rademakers, J. (2013): "The importance of patient-centered care for various patient groups". In: *Patient Education and Counseling*, 90 (3), pp. 405–410.

Elo, S./Kyngas, H. (2008): "The qualitative content analysis process". In: *Journal of Advanced Nursing*, 62 (1), pp. 107–15.

Ericsson, K. A./Simon, H. A. (1980): "Verbal reports as data". In: P*sychological Review*, 87 (3), pp. 215–251.

Frosch, D. L. (2015): "Patient-reported Outcomes as a Measure of Healthcare Quality". In: *Journal of General internal medicine*, 30 (10), pp. 1383–1384.

Lazar, E./Fleischut, P./Regan, B. K. (2013): "Quality Measurement in Healthcare". In: *Annual Review of Medicine*, 64 (1), pp. 485–496.

Lincoln, Y. S./Guba, E. G. (1985): *Naturalistic inquiry* (Vol. 75): Sage.

McKelvey, M. L./Hux, K./Dietz, A./Beukelman, D. (2010): "Impact of personal relevance and contextualization on wordpicture natching by people with aphasia". In: *American Journal of Speech and Language Pathology*, 19, pp. 22–33.

Poulson, D./Ashby, M./Richardson, S. (1996): *Userfit. A practical handbook on user centered design for Assistive Technology*. Brussels: ECSC-EC-EAEC.

National Quality forum. Available at: http://www.qualityforum.org/Patient-Reported Outcomes.aspx

Simpelaere, I. S./ban Nuffelen, G./de Bodt, M./Vanderwegen, J./Handen, T. (2017): "Validation of the Dutch version of the Swallowing Quality-of-Life Questionnaire (DSWAL-Qol) and adjused DSWAL-Qol (aDSWAL-QoL) using item analysis with the Rasch model: a pilot study". In: *Health and Quality of Life Outcomes*, 15 (1), pp. 66–82.

Stans, S./Dalemans, R./de Witte, L./Beurskens, A. (2013): "Challenges in the communication between 'communication vulnerable' people and their social environment: an exploratory qualitative study". In: *Patient Education Counseling*, 92 (3), pp. 302–12.

Swinburn, K./Best, W./Beeke, S./Cruice, M./Smith, L./Willis, E.P./ Ledingham, K./Sweeney, J./McVicker, S. J. (2018): "A concise patient reported outcome measure for people with aphasie: the aphasis impact questionnaire 21". In: *Aphasiology*, 33 (9), pp. 1035–1060.

Taylor, S./Guirguis, M./Raney, E. M. (2019): "Can Patients and Families Read the Questionnaires for Patient-related Outcome Measures?" In: *Journal of Pediatric Orthopaedics*, 39 (5): e397–401.

van Someren, M./Barnard, Y./Sandberg, J. (1994): *The think aloud method: A practical guide to modelling cognitive processes*. London: American Press.

Vas, A./Woods, A./Keebler, M./Spees, S. (2020): "SMART Program in Chronic Stroke". In: *Annals of International Occupational Therapy*, 3 (3), pp. 109–118. doi:doi: 10.3928/24761222-20200116-03

de Vet, H./Terwee, C.B./Mokkink, L.B./Knol, D.L. (2011): *Measurement in Medicine: A practical guide*. Cambridge University Press.

Wallace, S. E./Hux, K./Beukelman, D.R. (2010): "Navigation of a dynamic screen AAC interface by survivors of severe traumatic brain injury". In: *Augmentative and Alternative Communication*, 26 (4), pp. 242–254.

Wielaert, S. M./El Hachioui, H./van der Meulen, A.C./Neijenhuis, C.A.M. (2018). *AIQ-NL concept version*. Internal report.

Wilkinson, K. M./Light, J. (2011): "Preliminary investigation of visual attention to human figures in photographs: Potential considerations for the design of aided AAC visual scene displays". In: *Journal of Speech, language and hearing research*, 54 (6), pp. 1644–1657.

Nicola Häberle

Accessibility as a tool for health-literate organizations

Communication, access and navigation in organizational health literacy models and questionnaires

1 Introduction

The health care system in Germany is constantly shaped by an ongoing differentiation and more specialized health care. Patients, insured persons, and relatives are faced with increasingly complex requirements and a large variety of information possibilities. Accessibility in health care organizations is an elementary component for enabling participation, providing access, and enabling individuals to act on their own. In this context, research is gaining more and more insights into the extent to which promoting organizational health literacy can help improve communication, access, and navigation (Lubasch et al. 2021: 12646). Organizational health literacy (OHL) is demonstrated when health literacy is effectively embedded in organizational action. Bitzer and Sørensen (2018: 759) state that health care institutions that act appropriately with regard to the health literacy of clients and their individual abilities and skills, have organizational health literacy. Individual health literacy is thus context-dependent, i.e. whether and to what extent individuals can find their way in health care institutions must always be interpreted against the background of the concrete organizational conditions (Bitzer/Sørensen 2018: 755). Bitzer and Ernstmann (2019: 1) take up the definition from the U.S. Department of Health & Human Services (CDC 2021: 1), noting that competencies are latent constructs that manifest when they are needed. Therefore, they postulate with the following definition: "Health literacy is the degree to which individuals are enabled by the educational, social and/or health care system to find, process and understand health information relevant for appropriate health-related decisions" (Bitzer/Ernstmann 2019: 1).

In a position paper of the Health Literacy Network Germany (DNGK e.V.), Schaefer, Bitzer, and Dierks (2019: 2) differentiate those health-related decisions concerning the "individual values, goals and circumstances of citizens and patients, even if these decisions do not aim at the best medical outcome or contradict generally recognized, also evidence-based recommendations after well-founded consideration". In this context, Meggetto et al. (2017: 21) have highlighted in a systematic review that there are 19 different OHL terms or phrases to describe OHL and outlined how they can be understood and used. The importance of communication, access and navigation is evident in many terminologies (Meggetto et al. 2017: 21). Examples that illustrate this point particularly well are defined under the terms "Health literacy practice/s", "Health literacy environment", "Health literacy responsive/ness", "Health literacy systems level infrastructure" and "Improving health literacy in services", that "training and experience in communication, written information design, working with vulnerable populations, access and navigation of services and the service system; readability of forms, brochures and information" are a definition of terminologies aimed at describing the developments of the health literacy system (Megetto 2017: 23).

Farmanova et al. (2018: 1) also examined OHL guidelines. In their systematic literature review, the authors found that of 48 included publications, all addressed the topics of communication as well as access and navigation and that the workforce plays an important role not only in health care but also in the creation of a health-literate environment (Farmanova et al. 2018: 6). Furthermore, leadership was crucial in integrating health literacy into an organization's vision, mission, and strategic planning (Farmanova et al. 2008: 6). Analysing theoretical frames for OHL and OHL measuring tools, the following will highlight the elements "communication", "access", and "navigation".

2 Organizational health literacy: Theoretical framing and an overview of features of accessible communication

A model that characterizes individual health literacy as a dynamic concept and depicts the efforts of organizations to promote health literacy was developed by Bitzer and Sørensen (2018: 756). The authors state that the better the structures and processes of health care and the professionals acting within them, the more likely it is that health literacy will be achieved (Bitzer/Sørensen, 2018: 755). For this purpose, Bitzer and Sørensen (2018: 755) have developed a model that illuminates health literacy in the interaction of individuals with the health care system. This is presented as a self-generated, adapted model in Figure 1, with responsivity as the basis. The inner circle addresses the individual level of health literacy to be able to make health-related decisions. The outer, connecting circles target the organizational level with organizations directing their efforts at providing health-related information and services to promote the health literacy of their users. Bitzer and Sørensen (2018: 755) and Dodson et al. (2015: 13) show that systems and institutions, as well as facilities, are required to design and provide health information, sufficient resources, and support as well as the appropriate environment in such a way that they can be comparably accessed and used by all individuals with different levels of health literacy.

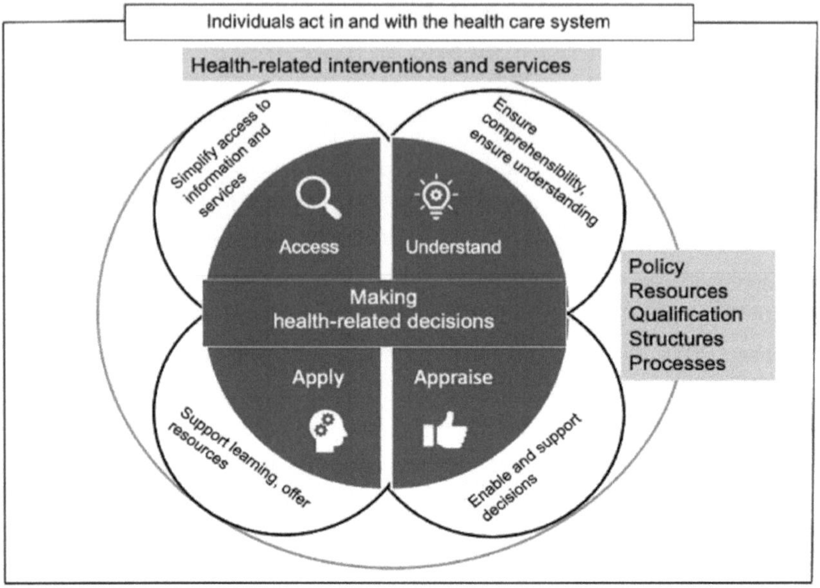

Figure 1: Own illustration based on Bitzer and Sørensen (2018: 756)

In this context, the Hildesheim Steps: "Hildesheimer Treppe", the Hildesheim school's accessible communication model for the comprehensibility of texts by the Research Centre for Easy Language (in German: Forschungsstelle Leichte Sprache, 2020: 15) can be linked to Figure 1. Central to this are the elements "understanding" and "appraising", which are also used in the model by the Forschungsstelle Leichte Sprache (2020: 15). The authors (Forschungsstelle Leichte Sprache 2020: 15) state that users can only act on the basis of texts that they can first find, perceive and thus comprehend. Subsequently, the texts are linked to previous knowledge and must correspond to the user's expectations and thus be accepted before the user can proceed to action (Forschungsstelle Leichte Sprache 2020: 15, Maaß 2020: 26). Especially for users with hearing or visual impairments, organizations can offer information in audiovisual forms with subtitles or sign language. In the following chapter, the concept of organizational health literacy with the 10 attributes will be discussed in more detail and options will be presented as to how organizations can "make it easier for people to navigate, understand, and use information and services" (Brach 2012: 1).

3 Improving organizational health literacy: 10 Attributes of health-literate health care organizations

A globally recognized and fundamental concept that characterizes health-literate organizations was developed in the USA by the Institute of Medicine (IOM) of the National Academy of Science in 2012 (Brach et al. 2012: 1–27). It was published as a discussion paper and states that a health-literate organization helps all people, including those with low health literacy levels, to obtain health-related and easily understandable information that they need for their individual decision-making (Brach et al. 2012: 2). The concept was predominantly developed for facilities involved in the provision of health services such as hospitals and rehabilitation centres or pharmacies and surgeries (Brach et al. 2012: 2). With regard to content, the concept consists of 10 attributes that should serve as a guide for the facilities and should be used to improve the environment (ibid.). To facilitate their use in practice, the authors have written implementation strategies for organizations promoting health literacy (ibid.). Table 1 shows the 10 attributes, which have also been adapted for the WHO Europe report "Health Literacy – The Solid Facts" (Kickbusch et al. 2013: 31–32).

1	Has leadership that makes health literacy integral to its mission, structure and operations	• Develops and implements policies and standards • Sets goals for improving health literacy improvement, establishes accountability and provides incentives • Allocates fiscal and human resources • Redesigns systems and physical space
2	Integrates health literacy into planning, evaluation measures, patient safety and quality improvement	• Conducts health literacy organizational assessments • Assesses the impact of policies and programs on individuals with limited health literacy • Factors health literacy into all patient safety plans

3	Prepares the workforce to be health literate and monitors progress.	• Hires diverse staff with expertise in health literacy • Sets goals for training staff at all levels
4	Includes populations served in designing, implementing and evaluating health information and services	• Includes individuals who are adult learners or have limited health literacy • Obtains feedback on health information and services from individuals who use them
5	Meets the needs of populations with a range of health literacy skills while avoiding stigmatization	• Adopts universal precautions for health literacy, such as offering everyone help with health literacy tasks • Allocates resources proportionate to the concentration of individuals with limited health literacy
6	Uses health literacy strategies in interpersonal communication and confirms understanding at all points of contact	• Confirms understanding (such as using the teach-back, show-me or chunk-and check methods) • Secures language assistance for speakers of languages other than the dominant language • Limits to two to three messages at a time • Uses easily understood symbols in way-finding signage
7	Provides easy access to health information and services and navigation assistance	• Makes electronic patient portals user-centered and provides training on how to use them • Facilitates scheduling appointments with other services
8	Designs and distributes print, audiovisual and social media content that is easy to understand and act on	• Involves diverse audiences, including those with limited health literacy, in development and rigorous user testing • Uses a quality translation process to produce materials in languages other than the dominant language

9	Addresses health literacy in high-risk situations, including care transitions and communication about medicines	• Gives priority to high-risk situations (such as informed consent for surgery and other invasive procedures) • Emphasizes high-risk topics (such as conditions that require extensive self-management)
10	Communicates clearly what health plans cover and what individuals will have to pay for services	• Provides easy-to-understand descriptions of health insurance policies • Communicates the out-of-pocket costs for health care services before they are delivered

Table 1: 10 Attributes of Health-Literate Health Care Organizations (Brach et al. 2012: 3)

3.1 Organizational health literacy: Changing perspectives and creating more accessibility

If the 10 attributes of health literacy promoting health care institutions are related to the hospital setting, it can be seen that communication, navigation, and access play an important role. Therefore, the following chapter shows a further description of the 10 attributes according to Brach et al. (2012: 3–19).

Attribute 1: Leadership promotes health literacy

The leadership of a hospital advocates health literacy as a core value of its mission statement, structures, and processes. Accordingly, employees who promote health literacy need leaders who present health literacy as a significant characteristic.

To be considered a health literacy-promoting organization, not only individual projects for the development of health literacy should be internalized, but rather health literacy should be consolidated as a central value system in the organization.

An organization and its culture are shaped by managers, which makes a health literacy-promoting attitude indispensable in order to take all employees with them (Schyve 2017: 2). In particular, leaders should communicate transparent guidelines and forms to employees and society. Leaders of a hospital that promote health literacy know the importance of communication and emphasize the health-competent rules of communication. Communication should be characterized by appreciation. Continuous evaluations should also be carried out to show where the organization and its individual employees can be assessed and which criteria need to be changed or adapted to move closer to the goals (Brach et al. 2012: 5–6).

Attribute 2: Health literacy and its integration in organizational processes

A hospital that promotes health literacy aligns strategic planning, evaluation measures, patient safety, and quality development in terms of health literacy; these factors describe the second attribute.

To fulfil the status of a health literacy promoting organization, health literacy must be integrated into all services, strategic and operational planning. Initiatives to promote health literacy must be created and evaluated at predetermined intervals (Brach et al. 2012: 6–7). For this purpose, indicators and measurement methods should be created and applied that enable valid and reliable measurements. Quality assurance is a basic requirement for health literacy promoting organizations. Therefore, quality development is important and patient well-being measures are used. The survey materials created for this purpose, e.g. questionnaires, must be formulated in a comprehensible way and provide opportunities and assistance to allow for further inquiries (Brach et al. 2012: 8). Communication mistakes are always documented to analyse causes and to identify systematic faults so that action can be taken. An example of a learning and reporting system in hospitals in Germany is CIRS (Critical Incident Reporting System), which is used for anonymous reporting of critical incidents as well as near misses (Bundesärztekammer 2022).

Attribute 3: Promotion of health literacy among employees

Institutions that improve health literacy assign a high relevance to staff training in the area of health literacy, which is explained in this third attribute. A culture can only be developed through comprehensive training, whereby a common goal, such as adapted communication, can be achieved. The target group for training in a hospital should not only be medical staff but also employees who represent the organization externally, e.g. reception staff. They need special didactic training to effectively inform and support patients. It is also beneficial for employees who are not in direct contact with patients, such as management staff, to take part in training courses in order to be aware of issues related to the promotion of health literacy and its further developments (Coleman 2011: 70). In addition, the group of new employees in a hospital must already be informed in introductory events about the purpose of health literacy improvement measures of the organization. At regular intervals, the health literacy skills of the employees are evaluated and those who need further training receive educational measures, the effects of which are then checked again (Brach et al. 2012: 8–9).

Attribute 4: Participation and cooperation of service users

Concerning practice, it can be stated that target group representatives such as patients in hospitals are unfortunately very rarely or not at all involved in the development and design of information and services (Münch/Dierks 2017: 72, Kowalski et al. 2015: 4). The perspectives of all stakeholders, especially those of people with low health literacy, are necessary when it comes to planning and developing programmes as well as materials to further develop health literacy. With the inclusion of the target group, both sides – organization and individuals – can benefit. On the one hand, the needs of the patients can be better integrated into the processes and structures of the organization, and on the other hand, the patients can better understand the whole organization with its processes and thus use the services more appropriately (Neuhauser et al. 2009: 2188). In a hospital it is therefore important that target group representatives are included in the advisory bodies as well as in the decision-making bodies (Brach et al. 2012: 9–10).

Attribute 5: Needs-oriented measures

As already mentioned in Chapter 2 with Figure 1 and in connection with the Hildesheim school's accessible communication model (Forschungsstelle Leichte Sprache 2020: 15), health literacy improving hospitals respond to each individual and make sure that the information is understood by the patients, e.g. with the help of audio-visual media. A health literacy improving organization strives to give priority to those individuals who have difficulties in understanding and navigating the information (Brach et al. 2012: 10–11). Additional support is provided by the organization, e.g. case managers assist with insurance matters. In the hospital setting, patient navigators, patient advocates or health educators can also be used (Brega et al. 2015: 35).

Attribute 6: Effective communication

Language barriers are a major challenge for quality assurance in health care. The less understanding of health and knowledge patients have, the more difficult it is to communicate (Logan 2017: 96, Schillinger et al. 2004: 315, Schillinger 2021: e233, Vernon et al. 2007: 2). People with low health literacy are mainly ashamed and consequently ask fewer questions or queries to health care providers (Schillinger et al. 2004: 315). If patients also have lower language skills, communication becomes even more difficult (Schenker et al. 2010: 224). The purpose of interventions is therefore to effectively promote two-way communication; various methods can be used to achieve this (Baker et al. 2011: 73). On the other hand, a trained and active staff team is also important. However, to help and support patients in their daily clinical routine, comprehensive communication structures, and patterns must be created. Clear communication is important, regardless of whether it is about directions or making an appointment.

Attribute 7: Providing information and enabling easy access

To make it easier for patients and visitors to find health information and services, targeted navigation measures are needed at the organizational level.

In health literacy improving organizations, it is important that more emphasis is placed on a user-friendly design that patients and citizens, as well as staff, can relate to.

In organizations that promote health literacy, attention is paid not only to an improved signage system and the structural design but also to the transmission of information by the staff (Groene/Rudd 2013: 227). Staff should provide visitors and patients with precise information and help them to find their way around the organization.

Many people are often overwhelmed by the amount of health information available. They often have little or no idea what to do with the amount of information available, which creates problems for them (Schaeffer et al. 2021: 58). This is becoming more and more of a challenge with an increasing amount of misinformation (Schaeffer et al. 2021: 3). In organizations that improve health literacy, these people should, on the one hand, receive support from the staff but on the other hand, they should also receive comprehensible information via electronic media (Lázaro Gutiérrez 2017: 140, Maaß/Hernández Garrido 2020: 131). Younger people in particular are increasingly using the internet for information (Schaeffer et al. 2021: 66). Both personal information, as well as educational content on health topics, can be accessed there; furthermore, it is possible to exchange information with other health care providers and to ask questions (anonymously) (Brach et al. 2012: 12–14).

As the Health Literacy Survey Germany 2 (HLS-Ger 2) on the health literacy of the population in Germany shows, it is difficult for many people to judge whether the information found on the internet is trustworthy and whether there is commercial interest behind the information (Schaeffer et al. 2021: 69). This underlines the need for reliable independent and evidence-based health information like informedhealth.org, which is why it is important for health literate institutions to place more emphasis on a user-friendly design that patients, but also staff, can relate to.

Health information in Easy and Plain Language is of equally high importance because, according to results of the LEO study from 2018, around 6.2 million adults aged 18–64 have low literacy skills, equivalent to alpha level 1–3 (Grotlüschen et al. 2019: 5). This corresponds to a share of 12.1 percent of the population in this age group. Combined with employment, the LEO study presents a result of 62.3 percent of all low-literate adults (Grotlüschen et al. 2019: 12). In summary, low literalization means that a person can read and write German up to the level of simple and shorter sentences, but fails at the level of connected texts (Grotlüschen/Buddeberg 2019: 343). Therefore, hospitals that improve health literacy create materials that are easy to understand and comprehensible for the users (Brach et al. 2012: 12–13). Against this background, reference can be made again to Figure 1, whereby health literacy promoting hospitals also support "understanding" with their structures and processes as well as qualifications.

Attribute 8: Media diversity

A health literacy promoting institution uses media diversity to ensure the understanding of the target group. If the current materials are not user-friendly, new materials are developed and designed (Brach et al 2012: 14). This is the responsibility of health literacy organizations and their experts.

Personal contact and training of patients are essential in health literacy organizations along with additional information materials. The written materials should be simply formulated and written in short sentences. Some tools can be used to develop easy-to-read materials in print and digital formats, such as the English-language Toolkit for Making Written Material Clear and Effective (Centers for Disease Control and Prevention 2020: 1) or Clear & Simple: Developing Effective Print Materials for Low-literate Readers (National Institutes of Health: 2021: 1). Relating to this, initiatives and recommendations for the use of Easy Language also exist in German-speaking countries; one example is the Handbook for Easy Language, which outlines the rules and principles (Bredel/Maaß 2016).

It is also very important that multilingual materials are available in organizations. If these are not sufficient, interpreters who are familiar with the respective culture and mother tongue must be called in (Brach et al. 2012: 16). Different media should also be applied. After use, the efforts for media diversity are evaluated and revised at regular intervals using suitable instruments. The users are also integrated into the evaluation by filling out customer questionnaires on the existing materials and providing further suggestions and potential for improvement (Brach et al. 2012: 14–16).

Attribute 9: Health literacy in high-risk situations

In clinical settings, communication and understanding are very important in interpersonal relationships. When making risky decisions, a higher level of reassurance is sought to check whether patients have internalized the information. In hospitals, examples of this would be consents for surgeries, prescriptions for medicines, and their intervals, and forms or applications. To avoid miscommunication in sensitive situations, organizations that improve health literacy should implement standards and processes that ensure a higher level of safety (Brach et al. 2012: 16–17). The teach-back method can be used, whereby the information conveyed must be reproduced by the patients in their own words. The chunk and check technique is another instrument through which information is conveyed in small pieces and only continued after the interlocutor has reproduced the information in his or her own words (NHS Scotland 2022). True to patient safety, self-management of intake and medication safety must also be primarily improved. For this reason, organizations that improve health literacy attach importance to providing patients with personal information and support in the form of various aids (e.g. medication dispensers, dosage aids, etc.) to ensure that patients understand how to take their medication correctly (Brach et al. 2012: 17–18).

Attribute 10: Transparency of services

The aim of health-literate organizations is to provide information and contact details of insurance providers in order to help people making informed decisions. First and foremost, education about covered services and costs must take place at the point of service delivery i.e. at the health care organizations. Here, too, proper communication and understanding of the other party play a role that should not be neglected. For example, doctors should know which medicines are financed and which medicines require further authorization. Before patients give their consent to treatment, they must be informed about the risks, side effects, and costs involved (Brach et al. 2012: 18–19). Looking at the country of origin of this concept, the tenth attribute plays a major role in the United States of America due to the elucidation of forms of financing for self-payers. However, in Germany the health care system has different prerequisites, therefore, this attribute is not further relevant for the German-speaking region. It has also been neglected in further research on the status of organizational health literacy in German hospitals (Münch 2018: 37).

4 Measurement of organizational health literacy and its instruments using a toolbox

For the development and improvement of an organization in terms of health literacy with target group-specific interventions, a presentation and assessment of the current state are required. This can be done with the help of a written survey of the different actors. Currently, 150 measurement instruments are available internationally, which differ in terms of length (from 1–3 to 40 items), focus (general vs. disease-specific) as well as the type of application (written/online/oral) and the psychometric properties (Bitzer/Sørensen 2018: 756). Concerning organizational health literacy, two instruments have established themselves in the German-speaking area. The first instrument is the Vienna Model of Health Competence in Health Care Organizations by the Ludwig Boltzmann Institute Health Promotion Research (LBIHPR), which was developed in cooperation with the Austrian Network of Health Promoting Hospitals (ONGKG) (Dietscher et al. 2015a: 8) and the second instrument is the health literate health care organization 10-item questionnaire (HLHO-10) by Kowalski et al. (2015: 4).

In the Vienna Model of Health Competence in Health Care Organizations four objectives were targeted: *access to living and working in a hospital; treatment, care, and therapy; disease prevention and management;* and *health promotion and lifestyle development (*Dietscher et al. 2015a: 9). In addition to patients, other stakeholders such as staff and society were also focused on as a further target group. To operationalize health literacy (HL), 9 standards with a total of 22 sub-standards and 160 items were applied (see Table 2, Dietscher et al. 2015a: 11). As Bitzer and Sørensen (2018: 759) describe, the concept links the topics of organizational health literacy with quality management strategies. The implementation of the model was supported by the provision of a self-assessment tool and a toolbox, which can also be used for auditing (Dietscher et al. 2015a: 14).

<table>
<tr><th></th><th>Patients</th><th>Staff</th><th>Community</th><th>Organizational structures & process-capacities implementation</th></tr>
<tr><td>Domain 1
Access to, living & working in the organization</td><td colspan="3">Standard 4: Navigation assistance
4.1 Accessible contact via website and telephone
4.2 Provision of information relevant for arrival and hospital stay
4.3 Availability of support at main entrance
4.4 Clear and easy-to-understand navigation system
4.5 Free availability of health information for patients and visitors</td><td rowspan="4">Standard 1: Management policy and organizational structures
1.1 HL as corporate responsibility
1.2 Quality assurance of HL

Standard 2: Participative development of materials and services
2.1 Participation of patients
2.2 Participation of staff

Standard 9: Dissemination and further development
9.1 support of the dissemination and further development of health literacy</td></tr>
<tr><td>Domain 2
Diagnosis, treatment & care</td><td>Standard 5: HL in patient communication
5.1 in spoken communication
5.2 in written communication
5.3 support by language translators and interpreters
5.4 also in high-risk situations</td><td>Standard 3: Develop HL skills of staff for patient communication
3.1 for all situations that involve communication</td><td rowspan="2">Standard 8: Contribute to HL in the region
8.1: promotion of continuous and integrated care</td></tr>
<tr><td>Domain 3
Disease management & prevention</td><td>Standard 6: Promote HL of patients and relatives
6.1 for disease-specific self-management</td><td>Standard 7: Promote HL of staff
7.1 for the self-management of occupational health and safety risks</td></tr>
<tr><td>Domain 4
Healthy lifestyle development</td><td>Standard 6: Promote HL of patients and relatives
6.2 for healthy lifestyle development</td><td>Standard 7: Promote HL of staff HL
7.2 for healthy lifestyles</td><td>Standard 8: Contribute to HL in the region
8.2 contribution to public health within the realm of possibility</td></tr>
</table>

Table 2: Self-assessment tool following the Vienna-Health Literate Organisation model (Pelikan 2016: 13) (Author's own representation)

The Vienna Health Literate Organisation (V-HLO) Instrument was tested between October 2014 and March 2015 in 9 Austrian hospitals for comprehensibility, relevance, and feasibility as well as its usefulness for organizational diagnosis and basic applicability for benchmarking between organizations and organizational units (Dietscher et al. 2015a: 11). The comprehensibility of the standards, sub-standards and items was confirmed by the participants in the pilot survey, and suggestions for improvement were incorporated. The pilot institutions set up multi-professional teams to conduct the self-assessment in the best possible way.

The results of the pilot facilities show that no facility or standard achieved very good scores. The greatest potential for improvement was found in Standard 2 (Develop and evaluate materials and services in a participatory manner), Standard 3 (Qualify staff for health literate communication with patients), and Standard 1 (Establish management principles and corporate structure for health literacy). The best results were achieved for Standard 4 (create a supportive environment – navigation aids and access to health information) and Standard 7 (improve the health literacy of staff) (Dietscher et al. 2015b: 7).

Dietscher et al. (2015a: 49) point out which measures can be implemented as a result of the pilot study and with regards to the further development of accessibility, the Vienna model also shows different approaches. For example, Standard 3 considers health literacy communication with patients as oral communication with the methods "Ask me Three" and "Teach back". "Ask me Three" is a method that encourages patients and their families to ask three specific questions of their providers to better understand their health conditions and what they need to do to stay healthy. The questions are: What is my main problem? What do I need to do? Why is it important for me to do this? In Germany, there are also campaigns such as the Health Network for Billstedt and Horn. With their campaign "3 Fragen für Ihre Gesundheit" they want to activate patients and improve their communicative skills (Gesundheit für Billstedt/Horn UG 2017).

In Standard 4, Dietscher et al. (2015a: 24) suggest that the organization should enable accessible initial contact via the Internet and telephone; for example, the website should be found in Plain Language with clear and simple text. Moreover, native-language communication is also addressed by the

Vienna model regarding telephone or video communication or in signposting and signage (Standard 4, Dietscher et al. 2015a: 29). Furthermore, the authors demonstrate that an organization that promotes health literacy asks for and takes into account different communication needs (e.g., language). In addition, adequately trained translators are always consulted if necessary, and when communicating with non-native speakers, employees should take this into account and for example speak more slowly (Dietscher et al. 2015a: 50).

Another self-assessment instrument that can be classified as a reliable and valid measurement tool is the health literate health care organization 10-item questionnaire (HLHO-10) by Kowalski et al. (2015: 4). Based on the 10 attributes of a health literate organization according to Brach et al. (2012: 3) (see Table 1), a questionnaire with 10 items was developed based on a literature review, an expert workshop, and a focus group discussion as well as qualitative interviews. In the validation study, 51 breast cancer centres were included and the questionnaire achieved acceptable to good properties in terms of psychometric properties. As the authors describe, there are two ways to use the HLHO-10 instrument (Kowalski et al. 2015: 6). The first way is to network the instrument in research to demonstrate the extent to which healthcare organizations are able to respond to the health literacy of patients and citizens (Kowalski et al. 2015: 8). The second way shows that the HLHO-10 can be used as a self-assessment tool to identify needs in order to better respond to patients' health literacy (Kowalski et al. 2015: 8).

This instrument is widely used in research. The HLHO-10 has already been used in a survey on patient orientation in the health care region of Cologne (SOPHIA) (Hower et al. 2019: 43). This survey showed that of the 237 participating facilities, the greatest needs were assessed in the inclusion of patients, in the development of health information as well as in individualized health information in different languages, font sizes with Braille and further efforts (Hower et al. 2019: 4). The facilities in the Cologne region also assess a need for patient orientation in the development of health information. Moreover, they still see the potential to provide information for different patients via different media such as picture stories or DVDs, but also three-dimensional models.

The training of staff was also emphasized, which is still needed on the topic of health literacy (Hower et al. 2019: 4).

Furthermore, the HLHO-10 is also used in a German university hospital, where it is interesting to see whether the information on organizational health literacy is similar across departments, occupational groups, and patient groups (Lubasch et al. 2021: 1).

5 Conclusion

Health literacy is of great importance in the health system and health care organizations and can create opportunities to expand accessibility in addressing communication, access, and navigation as the 10 attributes of health literate organizations show. It can also be emphasized that improving health literacy in organizations can contribute to improving the quality of treatment outcomes (Dietscher et al. 2015a: 7). In addition, various approaches analyse and highlight the need for development of health literacy in healthcare institutions (Lubasch et al. 2021: 1, Hower et al. 2019: 2). As the previous chapters show, there are existing concepts, instruments, and practical experiences that act as organizational diagnoses or also implementation tools (Kowalski et al. 2015: 6, Dietscher et al. 2015a: 11).

The National Action Plan on Health Literacy (NAP) in Germany also focuses on the topic, which emphasizes the responsibility of the organizations (Schaeffer et al. 2018: 38). In Strategy Paper #4 on Recommendations 6–10 of the National Action Plan in Germany, five strategic proposals are discussed that address navigation in the health care system, as well as the communication competence of health care professionals and the user-friendly design of health information or patient participation (Schmidt-Kaehler et al. 2019: 4). In this context, it can be seen that accessibility plays a decisive role, as is shown for example in the user-oriented development of information. Thus, an “interpreter service” is needed in a double sense, so that vulnerable target groups are more comprehensively encountered and cultural diversity is taken into account accordingly (Schmidt-Kaehler et al. 2019: 7).

In Germany, the Health Literacy Network Germany has joined forces to develop, evaluate and disseminate methods and concepts for promoting health literacy. One focus is on organizational health literacy and there is a working group on this topic. For the network and as a result of this working group, the authors Schaefer, Bitzer, and Dierks (2019: 7) have set up measures to strengthen organizational health literacy, which are intended to advance organizational health literacy in the prevailing health system. These are presented below.

The collection and documentation of already existing initiatives and instruments ("a kind of mapping") are reported to be able to specifically record and direct needs as well as ongoing or completed projects and programs (Schaefer et al. 2019: 7).

In addition, the collection of examples of successful implementation of organizational health literacy and analysis of facilitating factors and barriers, i.e. a collection of best practices, is declared desirable (Schaefer et al. 2019: 7).

Improving the visibility and implementation of reliable health information in the sense of "good health information practice" is also necessary, as is the adaptation or development of criteria for organizational health literacy for health care institutions (Schaefer et al. 2019: 7). Schaefer, Bitzer, and Dierks (2019: 8) also write about the (further) development of standards for health-competent organizations and the development of proposals and measures for implementation.

Networking of the institutions affected by the promotion of organizational health literacy is considered useful, as is the creation of framework conditions in the health system that are oriented towards the common good and enable all health professionals to actively promote the health literacy of their addressees through information, advice, education, and guidance (Schaefer et al. 2019: 8). Finally, the authors emphasize the development and implementation of strategies to promote the health and user competence of the different user groups in the health care system, taking into account vulnerable groups such as people with special needs, with low socio-cultural and economic resources, people with a migration background, people with chronic diseases, disabilities or in old age (Schaefer et al. 2019: 8).

In conclusion, the concept of organizational health literacy describes different possibilities for the micro/meso and macro levels of the health system and can help to improve communication, access and navigation for users. Furthermore, measurement tools already exist that enable organizations to identify the fields of action that need to be addressed with regard to the improvement of organizational health literacy. It is important that health care organizations recognise their mission in this respect and, as shown in Figure 1, that structures and processes need to be adapted in such a way that they enable all users to make appropriate health-related decisions.

Literature

Baker, David W./DeWalt, Darren A./Schillinger, Dean/Hawk, Victoria/Ruo, Bernice/Bibbins-Domingo, Kirsten/Weinberger, Morris/Macabasco-O'Connell, Aurelia/Pignone, Michael (2011): "'Teach to goal': Theory and design principles of an intervention to improve heart failure self-management skills of patients with low health literacy." In: *Journal of Health Communication, 16 Suppl 3*, pp. 73–88.

Bitzer, Eva Maria/Ernstmann, Nicole (2019): "Vorschlag für eine erweiterte Definition von Health Literacy". In: https://dngk.de/gesundheitskompetenz/definition-health-literacy-august-2019/ (letzter Zugriff: 20.08.2021).

Bitzer, Eva Maria/Sørensen, Kristine (2018): "Gesundheitskompetenz – Health Literacy." In: *Gesundheitswesen (Bundesverband der Ärzte des Öffentlichen Gesundheitsdienstes (Germany))*, 80 (8–09), pp. 754–766.

Brach, Cindy/Keller, Debra/Hernandez, Lyla/Baur, Cynthia/Parker, Ruth/Dreyer, Benard/Schyve, Paul/Lemerise, Andrew J./Schillinger, Dean (2012): *Ten Attributes of Health Literate Health Care Organizations.* NAM Perspectives, 02 (6).

Bredel, Ursula/Maaß, Christiane (2016): *Leichte Sprache: Theoretische Grundlagen, Orientierung für die Praxis. Sprache im Blick.* Dudenverlag.

Brega Angela G./Barnard, Juliana/Mabachi, Natabhona M./Weiss Barry D./DeWalt Darren A./Brach, Cindy/Cifuentes Maribel/Albright, Karin/West, David (2015): *AHRQ Health Literacy Universal Precautions Toolkit, Second Edition. Prepared by Colorado Health Outcomes Program, University of Colorado Anschutz Medical Campus under Contract No.*

HHSA290200710008, TO#10. Rockville, MD. Agency for Healthcare Research and Quality.

Bundesärztekammer (2022): "*CIRSmedical*". In: https://www.cirsmedical.de/ (letzter Zugriff: 21.05.2022)

Centers for Disease Control and Prevention (2021): "What Is Health Literacy?". In: https://www.cdc.gov/healthliteracy/learn/index.html#wnd (letzter Zugriff: 23.08.2021).

Centers for Medicare & Medicaid Services (2020): "Toolkit for Making Written Material Clear and Effective". In: https://www.cms.gov/utreach-and-Education/Outreach/WrittenMaterialsToolkit (letzter Zugriff: 23.08.2021).

Coleman, Clifford (2011): "Teaching health care professionals about health literacy: A review of the literature." In: *Nursing Outlook*, 59 (2), pp. 70–78.

Dietscher, Christina/Lorenc, Jakob/Pelikan, Jürgen (2015a): "Das Selbstbewertungs-Instrument zum Wiener Konzept Gesundheitskompetenter Krankenbehandlungsorganisationen (WKGKKO-I)." In: https://oepgk.at/wkgkko-1-selbstbewertungs-instrument/ (letzter Zugriff: 24.08.2021).

Dietscher, Christina/Lorenc, Jakob/Pelikan, Jürgen (2015b): "Toolbox 2015: zum Wiener Konzept Gesundheitskompetenter Krankenbehandlungsorganisationen (WKGKKO)." In: https://oepgk.at/wkgkko-toolbox-2015/ (letzter Zugriff: 24.08.2021).

Dodson Sarity/Good Suvajee/Osborne, Richard (2015): "Optimizing Health Literacy: Improving Health and Reducing Health Inequities." In: https://www.google.com/url?sa=t&rct=j&q=&esrc=s&source=web&cd=&ved=2ahUKEwjntrW_ycXzAVTA2MBHaM8AWUQFnoECBMQAQ&url=https%3A%2F%2Fapps.who.int%2Firis%2Fbitstream%2Fhandle%2F10665%2F205594%2FB5147.pdf%3Fsequence%3D1%26isAllowed%3Dy&usg=AOvVaw1rDg6OOSJ_QqonXhyBHMSL (letzter Zugriff: 24.08.2021).

Farmanova, Elina/Bonneville, Luc/Bouchard, Louise (2018): "Organizational Health Literacy: Review of Theories, Frameworks, Guides, and Implementation Issues". In: *Inquiry: A Journal of Medical Care Organization, Provision and Financing, 55*, 46958018757848.

Forschungsstelle Leichte Sprache (2020): *Erkenntnis und Transfer: Barrierefreie Kommunikation als gesellschaftliche Aufgabe und Gegenstand der Forschung*. In: https://www.uni-hildesheim.de/en/fb3/institute/institut-fuer-uebersetzungswissfachkommunikation/forschungsprojekte/leichtesprache/forschung/publikationen/ (letzter Zugriff: 21.05.2021).

Gesundheit für Billstedt/Horn UG. (2017): *Gesundheitskompetenz*. In: https://experten.gesundheit-bh.de/gesundheitskompetenz/ (letzter Zugriff: 21.05.2022)

Groene, Raluca O./Rudd, Rima E. (2013): "Results of a feasibility study to assess the health literacy environment: navigation, written, and oral communication in 10 hospitals in Catalonia, Spain". In: *Journal of Communication in Healthcare*, 4 (4), pp. 227–237.

Grotlüschen Anke/Buddeberg Klaus (2019): "Geringe Literalität unter Erwachsenen in Deutschland". In: Quenzel, Gudurn/Hurrelmann, Klaus (Hg.): *Handbuch Bildungsarmut*. Wiesbaden: Springer Fachmedien, pp. 341–361.

Hower, Kira/Poppe, Adriana/Vennedey, Vera/Hillen, Hendrik/Kuntz, Ludwig/Stock, Stephanie/Pfaff, Holger/Ansmann, Lena (2019): "Survey on Patient Orientation in Health and Social Care Organizations (SOPHIA). Fragebogen zur Patientenorientierung in Versorgungsorganisationen in der Stadt Köln: Kennzahlenhandbuch". In: http://www.imvr.de/de/forschung/projekte (letzter Zugriff: 26.08.2021).

Kickbusch, Ilona/Pelikan, Jürgen/Haslbeck, Jörg/Apfel, Franklin/Tsouros, Agis D. (2013): "Health Literacy. The Solid Facts" In: http://gbv.eblib.com/patron/FullRecord.aspx?p=1582975 (letzter Zugriff: 20.08.2021).

Kowalski, Christoph/Lee, Shoou-Yih D./Schmidt, Anna/Wesselmann, Simone/Wirtz, Markus A./Pfaff, Holger/Ernstmann, Nicole (2015): "The health literate health care organization 10 item questionnaire (HLHO-10): Development and validation". In: *BMC Health Services Research, 15*, p. 47.

Lázaro Gutiérrez, R. (2017): "Healthcare Videos Addressed to the Migrant Population: From Intercultural Mediation to Transcreation". In: *Revista De Lenguas Para Fines Específicos*, 23 (1), 140–162.

Logan, Robert A. (2017): "Seeking an Expanded, Multidimensional Conceptual Approach to Health Literacy and Health Disparities Research". In: *Studies in Health Technology and Informatics, 240*, pp. 96–123.

Lubasch, Johanna S./Voigt Barbarowicz, Mona/Ernstmann, Nicole/Kowalski, Christoph/Brütt, Anna Levke/Ansmann, Lena (2021). "Organizational Health Literacy in a Hospital-Insights on the Patients' Perspective". In: *International Journal of Environmental Research and Public Health, 18* (23).

Lubasch, Johanna S./Voigt-Barbarowicz, Mona/Lippke, Sonia/Wilde, Rudy L. de/Griesinger, Frank/Lazovic, Djordje/OcampoVillegas, Paloma C./Roeper, Julia/Salzmann, Daniela/Seeber, Gesine H./Torres-de-la-Roche, Luz-Angela/Weyhe, Dirk/Ansmann, Lena/Brütt, Anna L. (2021): "Improving professional health literacy in hospitals: Study protocol of a participatory codesign and implementation study". In: *BMJ Open*, *11* (8), e045835.

Maaß, Christiane (2020): *Easy Language – Plain Language – Easy Language Plus.* Frank & Timme.

Maaß, Christiane/Sergio Hernández Garrido (2020): "Easy and Plain Language in Audiovisual Translation". In Hansen-Schirra, Silvia/Maaß, Christiane (Ed.): *Easy Language Research: Text and User Perspectives.* (pp. 131–161). Frank & Timme.

Meggetto, Elizabeth/Ward, Bernadette/Isaccs, Anton (2017): "What's in a name? An overview of organisational health literacy terminology". In: *Australian Health Review: A Publication of the Australian Hospital Association*, *42* (1), pp. 21–30.

Münch, Inga/Dierks, Marie-Luise (2017): "Health Literate Organizations – ein Konzept für den deutschen stationären Sektor?" In: *Public Health Forum*, *25* (1), pp. 71–73.

Münch, Inga (2018): *Health Literate Organizations – ein Konzept für Einrichtungen der akutstationären Versorgung und der Rehabilitationseinrichtungen in Deutschland.* Dissertation. Medizinische Hochschule Hannover.

National Institutes of Health (2021): *Clear & Simple.* In: https://www.nih.gov/institutes-nih/nih-office-director/office-communications-public-liaison/clear-communication/clear-simple (letzter Zugriff: 23.08.2021).

Neuhauser, Linda/Rothschild, Beccah/Graham, Carrie/Ivey, Susan L./Konishi, Susana (2009): "Participatory design of mass health communication in three languages for seniors and people with disabilities on Medicaid". In: *American Journal of Public Health*, *99* (12), pp. 2188–2195.

NHS Scotland (2022): *Techniques.* In: https://www.healthliteracyplace.org.uk/toolkit/techniques/ (letzter Zugriff: 21.05.2022).

Pelikan, Jürgen (2016): "The Vienna model for health literate hospitals: engaging patients and caregivers". In: https://www.google.com/url?sa=t&rct=j&q=&esrc=

s&source=web&cd=&cad=rja&uact=8&ved=2ahUKEwjX_dux5cXzAhVS3qQKHW8VA6wQFnoECAYQAQ&url=https%3A%2F%2Fwww.bumc.bu.edu%2Fhealthliteracyconference%2Ffiles%2F2016%2F06%2FJurgen_Pelikan.pdf&usg=AOvVaw2rKcHgQjrFTiKNr6o6D0h9 (letzter Zugriff: 21.08.2021).

Schaefer, Corinna/Bitzer, Eva Maria/Dierks, Marie-Luise für den Vorstand des DNGK (2019): "Mehr Organisationale Gesundheitskompetenz in die Gesundheitsversorgung bringen! Ein Positionspapier des DNGK". In: https://dngk.de/gesundheitskompetenz/organisationale-gesundheitskompetenz-positionspapier-2019/ (letzter Zugriff: 20.08.2021).

Schaeffer, Doris/Berens, Eva-Maria/Gille, Svea/Griese, Lennert/Klinger, Julia/Sombre, Steffen de/Vogt, Dominique/Hurrelmann, Klaus (2021), "Gesundheitskompetenz der Bevölkerung in Deutschland vor und während der Corona Pandemie: Ergebnisse des HLS-GER 2". In: https://pub.uni-bielefeld.de/record/2950305 (letzter Zugriff: 23.08.2021).

Schaeffer, Doris/Hurrelmann, Klaus/Bauer, Ullrich/Kolpatzik, Kai (2018): *Nationaler Aktionsplan Gesundheitskompetenz: Die Gesundheitskompetenz in Deutschland stärken*. Berlin: KomPart.

Schenker, Yael/Karter, Andrew J./Schillinger, Dean/Warton, E. Margaret/Adler, Nancy E./Moffet, Howard H./Ahmed, Ameena T./Fernandez, Alicia (2010): "The impact of limited English proficiency and physician language concordance on reports of clinical interactions among patients with diabetes: The DISTANCE study". In: *Patient Education and Counseling, 81* (2), pp. 222–228.

Schillinger, Dean (2021): "Social Determinants, Health Literacy, and Disparities: Intersections and Controversies". In: *Health Literacy Research and Practice, 5* (3), e234-e243.

Schillinger, Dean/Bindman, Andrew/Wang, Frances/Stewart, Anita/Piette, John (2004): "Functional health literacy and the quality of physician-patient communication among diabetes patients". In: *Patient Education and Counseling, 52* (3), pp. 315–323.

Schmidt-Kaehler, Sebastian/Schaeffer, Doris/Hurrelmann, Klaus/Pelikan, Jürgen (2019): "*Strategiepapier #4 zu den Empfehlungen des Nationalen Aktionsplans. Gesundheitskompetenz als Standard auf allen Ebenen im*

Gesundheitssystem verankern". In: https://pub.uni-bielefeld.de/record/2935460 (letzter Zugriff: 23.08.2021).

SCHYVE, PAUL (2017): "Leadership in Healthcare Organizations: A Guide to Joint Commission Leadership Standards." In: https://www.google.com/url?sa=t&rct=j&q=&esrc=s&source=web&cd=&cad=rja&uact=8&ved=2ahUKEwjBxN79wsXzAhUT4OAKHU66AmUQFnoECAcQAQ&url=https%3A%2F%2Fnrchealth.com%2Fwp-content%2Fuploads%2F2017%2F06%2FWP_JC_Leadership-in-Healthcare-Organizations_Second_Schyve_Carr.pdf&usg=AOvVaw0RuqJqJqxEoWmNkBh0EJ30 (letzter Zugriff: 21.08.2021).

VERNON, JOHN/TRUJILLO, ANTONIO/ROSENBAUM, SARA/DEBUONO, BARBARA (2007): "*Low Health Literacy: Implications for National Health Policy*". In: https://hsrc.himmelfarb.gwu.edu/sphhs_policy_facpubs/172/ (letzter Zugriff: 23.08.2021).

Julian Hörner

Accessible and reliable health information on the internet

How we introduced Plain Language to apotheken-umschau.de – a project report[1]

1 Introduction

More than half of the German population experience considerable difficulties in locating, understanding, assessing and using health-related information. This finding of the Health Literacy Survey (HLS-GER) in Germany (Schaeffer et al. 2016)[2] and the resulting National Action Plan Health Literacy to promote health literacy in Germany (Schaeffer et al. 2018) has inspired us at Wort & Bild Verlag. After all, as Germany's leading health publisher, we consider it our responsibility to make reliable and helpful information on diseases, medications and preventive health care accessible to everyone with as few barriers as possible. In the Apotheken Umschau's online editorial team, our aim is to ensure that everyone who has difficulties navigating the maze of information, can find comprehensible information at apotheken-umschau.de (Presseportal

1 I would like to take this opportunity to express my heartfelt thanks to all those who have worked on this project in various roles to realize this special offer on our website:
First and foremost, my colleagues at Wort & Bild Verlag: Nina Buschek, Irmela Manus, Carolin Collin, Andreas Krenz, Andreas Kirchhammer and Ágota Vincze.
Then, of course, Janina Kröger, Christiane Maaß, Isabel Rink and their team of translators from the Research Center for Easy Language at the University of Hildesheim.
And last but not least, Dennis Ballwieser, who as the responsible editor-in-chief believed in this project from the very beginning and continues to support it.

2 From the follow-up study, HLS-GER 2, we now know that the health literacy of the population in Germany has actually deteriorated over the past seven years. At 58.8 percent, significantly more than half of the population has low health literacy (ct. Schaeffer et al. 2021).

2019, Oktober 3019) Confronted with these alarming study results, we began to ask ourselves: Are we really reaching the general public with our medical guides on the internet? How can we do better?

Amongst a few other approaches, we considered adding information boxes in Easy Language with brief summaries of our articles' central content. At a training course at the Academy of the Bavarian Press in March 2019, I wanted to acquire the necessary knowledge about the dos-and-don'ts of Easy Language in order to pass it on to my colleagues on the editorial team. During this two-day workshop, I quickly realized that the differences between texts in standard language and texts in Easy Language are quite considerable, and entails a real translation effort. We realized that we didn't have anyone on the editorial staff qualified to do this. Neither I nor my colleagues had the time to train as translators alongside our daily business. So if we wished to expand our service and create universal access to the linguistic content of our texts, we would have to hire a translation agency.

With this idea in mind, I approached my editor-in-chief Dennis Ballwieser and asked if we could commission such translations. He was immediately taken with the idea. After all, he was well aware of the problem of inadequate health literacy among the German population. As the person in charge of the largest consumer medium in the German-speaking area, he is constantly looking for ways to better reach our readers.

So we launched a test run. Initially, 10 texts were to be translated. If that went well, we could gradually have the entire lexical content of our medical guides translated. It was particularly important to us that the translation of our texts met the same standards that apply to our original texts: they would have to be scientifically sound, professionally verified and absolutely independent.

Fortunately, I quickly came across the Research Centre for Easy Language at the Institute for Translation Studies and Specialized Communication at the University of Hildesheim.

2 Initial strategic decisions: Balancing enhanced comprehensibility with acceptability

Together with our colleagues at the Research Centre, we first defined the primary target groups of our texts. In the process, we identified with the following groups of readers:

- People with cognitive impairments
- People with dementia-type illness
- People with visual and hearing impairments
- People with language impairments (e.g. after stroke)
- People with little knowledge of German or lack of language skills (e.g. due to migration experience)
- People with diverging educational opportunities

All these groups benefit greatly from texts in Easy Language. However, in the context of the website apotheken-umschau.de, Easy Language would probably have an acceptance problem due to some of its features like the ban on 3rd person pronouns, extensive explanations of words and concepts considered peripheral, or the rule to start a new line for each sentence (Maaß 2020). As one of the largest health portals in Germany, apotheken-umschau.de aims to reach the general public. Outside the context of public administration and social organizations, however, it is not (yet) a matter-of-course in German-speaking countries to encounter texts in Easy Language in online content. We were concerned that texts with these features would be rejected by the broad public and therefore contribute to stigmatization rather than inclusion. We wanted to avoid that at all costs. The translations should be as accessible, but at the same time as acceptable as possible. As Christiane Maaß points out in her volume Easy – Plain – Accessible: "The best offer isn't worth anything if it is not acceptable and therefore not used" (Maaß 2020: 11). For this reason, we decided to have the texts translated into Plain Language in consultation with the Research Centre for Easy Language. However, the linguistic ruleset of the texts was to be strongly oriented toward Plain Language and to be as perceptible and comprehensible as possible. The challenge in this context is to weight and balance perceptibility/comprehensibility on the one hand and acceptance/risk of stigmatization on the other (ibid.: 266). With our consent, the Research Centre for Easy Language executes our comprehensibility-enhanced texts as part of a research project. "This project is intended to shape guidelines for an enriched version of Easy Language defined as Easy Language Plus [...] At the same time, the project generates a corpus of health information texts in Easy Language Plus that is, to this day, the biggest in the German-speaking area: [...] text- and user-centred research is being conducted to explore perceptibility, comprehensibility, recall and acceptability of these texts in comparison with standard texts and texts that have the full range of Easy Language features." (ibid.: 264.; A more detailed description of the project's linguistic aspects are to be found in: ibid.: 262–275).

These evolving guidelines aim to bridge the gap between Easy Language and Plain Language as visualized in the figure below.

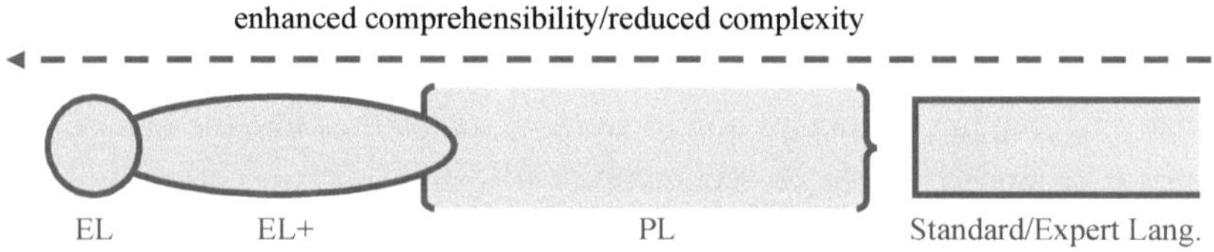

Figure 1: Easy Language – Easy Language Plus – Plain Language – Expert Language (Maaß 2020: 14)

Even though our translations are in fact texts in Easy Language Plus, we label our service as "Einfache Sprache" (Plain Language – PL). This term is recognized and reasonably well known. Accordingly, I will also use the term Plain Language throughout this paper, even though what is actually meant is Easy Language Plus. In this way, I would like to minimize possible confusion regarding the terminology.

3 Multi-stage translation process

Once we knew who we wanted to write for and how, we went on to define the corpus of text we wished to have translated. Our selection criteria for this were:

- Traffic:
  The articles to be translated should have a wide reach (measured in page impressions) in order for the translation to be noticed at all.
- Relevance:
  Which texts are relevant to the target audience according to the assessment of the medical colleagues?
- Currency of the guides:
  The guides to be translated should be as up-to-date as possible and should have been last updated no more than one year ago.[3]

All texts are scientifically reviewed twice: from a linguistic perspective by the Research Centre for Easy Language, and from a medical or pharmaceutical perspective by a member of the scientific editorial staff of Apotheken Umschau. Selected texts are sent to the Research Centre for Easy Language. The project lead there distributes the texts to a translator from their team. The translator produces a rough translation. This translation is first sent to a colleague at the Research Centre, who proofreads it and checks the language (dual control principle).

Only when the translation has been checked and is approved from a linguistic perspective, it is sent back to the editorial office at Apotheken Umschau. There, a member of our scientific editorial staff checks whether the medical information in the translation is still valid despite reduction of complexity and shortening. This step usually involves making the wording more precise so that it can be action-enabling for our readers in the medical sense. In the case of

3 Medical knowledge is in a constant state of flux. Accordingly, our editorial team relies on a regular update cycle for all medical advice texts. We do this regardless of the appearance of new medical treatment guidelines, which of course necessitate immediate updating of the corresponding health guides on our website.

translations into Plain Language, we therefore apply the same high standards that apply to all our publications and that make us outstanding in the field of German-language consumer media.

3.1 Structure of the guides

All our texts in Plain Language are kept as short as possible. On average, the print version comprises only three pages of Plain Language text (including images, where available). The texts follow a macrostructure that was developed by our partners at the Research Centre for Easy Language and which is based on the structure of the original texts. Ideally, the structure will follow the pattern below:

- What is XY?
- What happens with XY?
- How can you recognize XY?
- What are the causes of XY?
- What can you do about XY?
- Where can you get more information?

In the last section "Where can you get more information?", there is always a backlink that refers back to the original text. Of course, this structure is adapted to the respective requirements of the original text. We omit individual aspects or replace them with others if they do not make sense for the topic in question. Where necessary, we add thematic paragraphs. For example, in the guide on strokes, first aid measures are explicitly dealt with in a separate section of the text (Apotheken Umschau 2019, September 29). In texts on diagnostic methods, on the other hand, we tend to explain the procedure, the necessary preparations, or the risks associated with the respective measure (cf. Apotheken Umschau 2020, January 27). Advice texts on medicines and medicinal plants do not ask "What are the causes of XY?". In that case, the structure usually looks more like this:

- What is XY?
- How does XY work?
- What should you be aware of when using XY?
- What side effects are possible?
- What interactions are possible?
- Who should not use XY?
- Where can you get more information?

It is important to us that the texts always have an identical structure in order to enhance their perceptibility. The framing text modules (boxes) also contribute to this, labelling them as belonging to the Plain Language service. All texts are preceded by

- a standardized introductory sentence instead of a conventional article teaser: "Dieser Text informiert in Einfacher Sprache zum Thema: XY".[4]
- a table of content that allows users to jump directly to the relevant subheading (and return from there to the beginning of the text) via a jump mark navigation.[5]

At the end of the texts our readers will find two orange-coloured boxes:

- The first box is a teaser containing a link back to the landing page where all articles in Plain Language are listed.
- The second box bears the quality seal of the Research Centre for Easy Language and identifies this text as linguistically approved.

4 Translation by Julian Hörner: "This text informs in Plain Language about the topic: XY".

5 Thus, depending on the respective reading and comprehension skills or strategy, one can read the texts in their entirety or jump to the individual headings.

3.2 Layout of the guides

We have deliberately kept the layout of the texts in Plain Language simple and consistent with the aesthetics of the standard text. We do, however, use some comprehensibility-enhanced visual aids, following the recommendations of the Easy Language ruleset (Bredel/Maaß 2016). The amount of possible distractions from the text should be kept at a minimum: for example, we do not use large lead pictures or decorative images. We use photographs for illustration only in exceptional cases. Instead of photographs, we rely on infographics, as they present what is explained schematically and are easier to comprehend. In case of infographics being used to illustrate something, we make sure that they are particularly comprehensible by further reducing complexity where necessary (and possible).

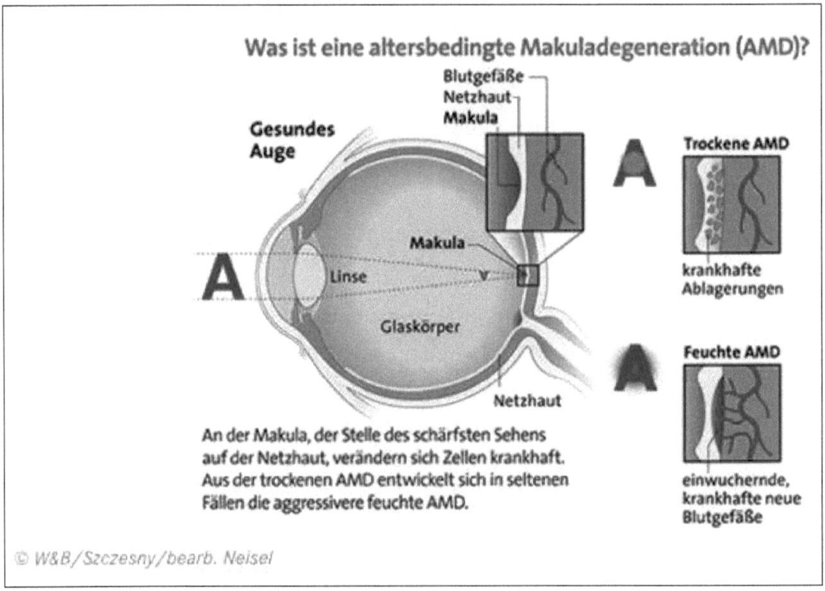

Figure 2A: Infographic of the original text explaining different variants of age-related macular degeneration (AMD) (Apotheken Umschau 2017, August 30)

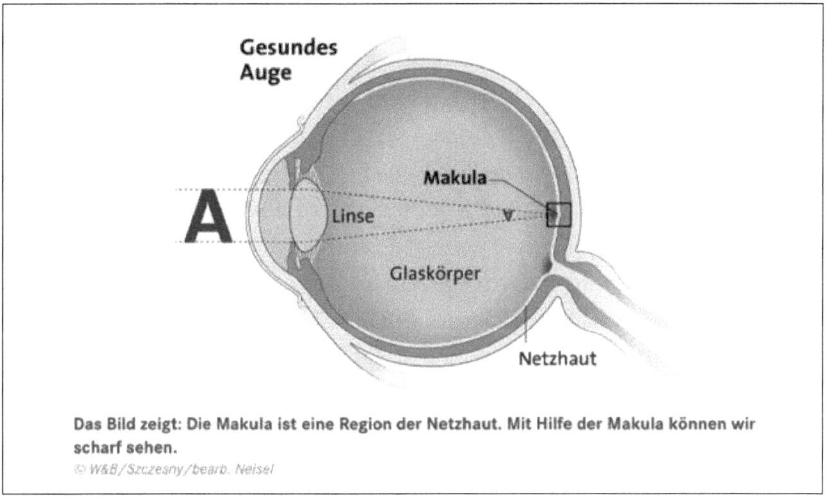

Figure 2B: Comprehensibility-enhanced infographic of the translation in Plain Language with less detail (ibid.: 2021, March 03)

For some articles, we use short explanatory videos of 60 to 90 seconds in length that briefly summarize the content of the text. These videos are subtitled and we pay particular attention to easy-to-understand presentations here, even if they are not produced specifically for our Plain Language service. As advised in the Easy Language ruleset, we use only boldface to highlight key terms and always use bullet points for lists. Only in special cases do we use coloured text boxes to highlight particularly critical information, such as warnings (cf. Apotheken Umschau 2020, February 06; Apotheken Umschau 2019, September 23a; Apotheken Umschau 2019, September 23b).

After consulting with the experts at the Research Centre for Easy Language, we decided to offer the entire range of Plain Language texts on our website free of advertising. Without the colourful advertising, we hope to ensure the best possible perceptibility of the texts – especially for people with visual impairments, dementia-type illness or cognitive impairments.

3.3 Where to find Plain Language texts on apotheken-umschau.de?

After receiving the first translations, we had to decide how to present them on our website. A landing page for a quick overview of all texts available in Plain Language was considered a good standard and therefore selected. All the Plain Language guides are collected on this landing page (https://www.apotheken-umschau.de/einfache-sprache). After a short address to the readers about the purpose of the articles in Plain Language, the reader finds an alphabetical listing of all translations on the landing page. We place selected articles prominently in front of this list with their own illustrated teaser boxes. Currently, these are articles on Covid-19.

It was important to us to anchor this landing page as high up in the website's navigation hierarchy as possible. In this way, we want to ensure that the guides can be found easily. If you visit apotheken-umschau.de, you will find the "Einfache Sprache" navigation node in the second navigation level directly under "Home", i.e. the homepage:

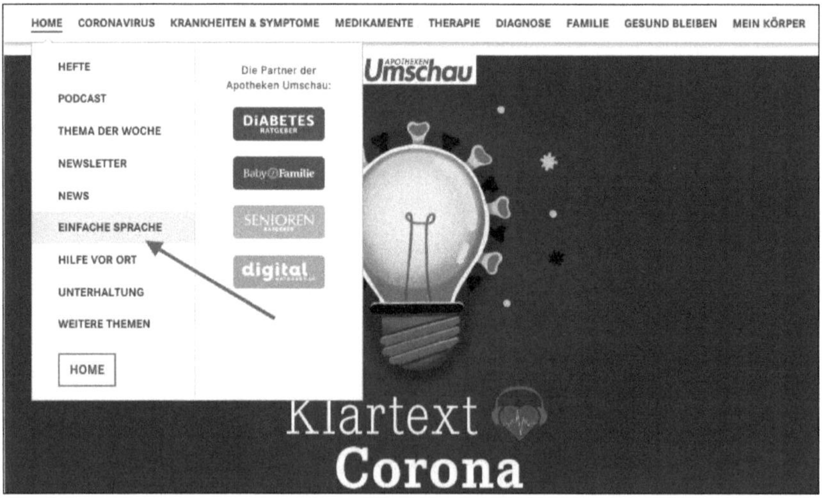

Figure 3A: Desktop view of the navigation bar of apotheken-umschau.de (Apotheken Umschau n.d.)

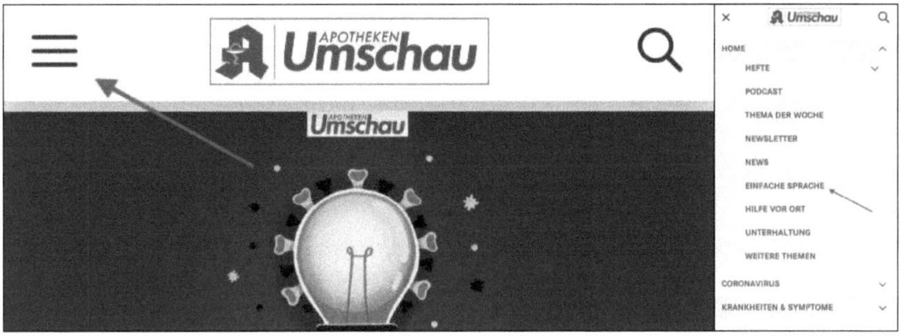

Figure 3B: On the left: In mobile view the navigation guide is located in the hamburger menu on the upper left corner (Apotheken Umschau n.d.).
Figure 3C: On the right: Opened navigation menu (Apotheken Umschau n.d.)

The landing page should not be the only entry into the cosmos of Plain Language on our site. My initial idea was that a button in the header should switch the whole site to the Plain Language version. This feature is quite common on the websites of German authorities or non-profit associations. We decided against it for two reasons:

1. Since we initially had only few translations, readers would have to be redirected to a landing page, a mission statement or the like too often. This would probably have put users off and jeopardized the acceptance of the entire service.
2. Such a feature would have deeply interfered with the basic functions of the website and would not have been possible with our CMS (Content Management System).

Instead, we decided to integrate the translations into the existing guides and to place them alongside the original texts as a kind of twin. We deliberately opted for a neutral presentation. In this way, we wanted to emphasize the seriousness of our service. The cartoon characters with the open book, so often found in the context of Plain/Easy Language, are perceived by many readers as stigmatizing, as the experts from the Research Centre for Easy Language assured us during the vote on our logo. In the layout of the original texts, we therefore placed a flag prominently and in the signal colour orange. It says

"Text in einfacher Sprache"[6]. Clicking on it takes readers to the corresponding translation in Plain Language:

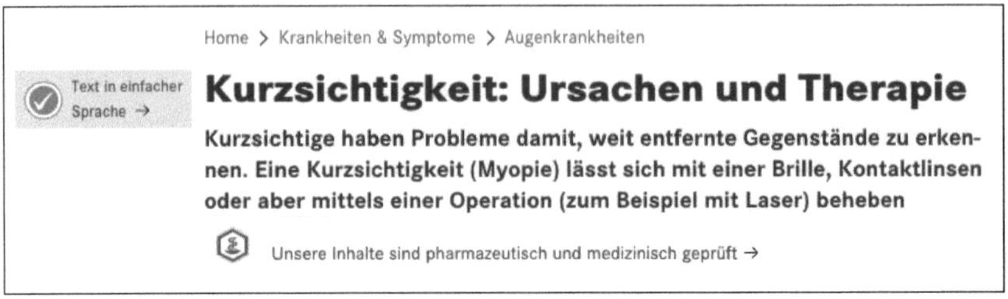

Figure 4A: Desktop view: Overview and teaser of one of our original texts with the striking mark that refers to the translation in Plain Language to the left of the headline (Apotheken Umschau 2019, July 08)

In mobile view we have implemented it correspondingly:

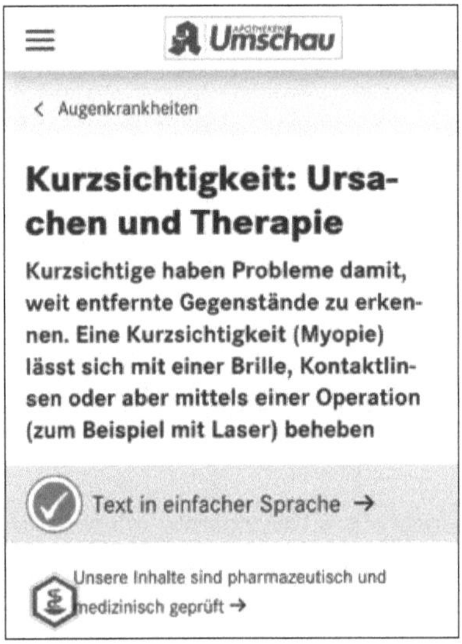

Figure 4B: Mobile view: Overview and teaser of one of our original texts with the striking mark that refers to the translation in Plain Language directly below the article teaser (Apotheken Umschau 2019, July 08)

6 Translation by Julian Hörner: "Text in Plain Language".

However, the prominent anchoring of the Plain Language texts in the layout of the original texts also led to discussions amongst the editorial staff. The reference to Plain Language at the very top, next to the headline, was considered too dominant by some colleagues. Their concern was that, placed so prominently, the mark could lead our readers away from the actual content. In addition, the orange colour of the button strays from the usual colour scheme of the apotheken-umschau.de portal, and the layout of the articles looks unstable if we place the button in the white space next to the headline in desktop view. In mobile view, we also waste too much space on the precious first screen, where the central content should be visible without scrolling.

Eventually we decided on this representation for the following reasons:

1. The orange of the button picks up on the orange of the quality seal of the Research Centre for Easy Language and is intended to label the translations as belonging to the original text, but as an independent service.
2. The maximum prominence of the location next to the headline (or directly below it, in mobile view) ensures that we reach as many potential readers as possible with this additional offer – the sooner they come across information that corresponds to their respective reading and comprehension skills, the greater the chance that they will also engage with the content provided.
3. The prominent location in the layout of the original texts has another effect: with regards to the general public, it gives visibility to our target group of people with communication impairments.
4. It is a token of apotheken-umschau.de's commitment to social inclusion.

The links of the orange buttons lead from the original texts to the translations. For our guides in Plain Language, we built a parallel link network of keyword links to relevant guides. This means that we do not link to our standard language guides, but only to our translations. Once readers are in the Plain Language area, they can find other Plain Language guides on the topics addressed. In this way, we enable them to research health topics independently within an accessible environment. This link network is constantly growing and densifying with every new translation published online. If we consider a non-PL guide or an external source to be indispensable, we provide the link with a corresponding note that this text is not written in Plain Language. The same applies in the case of the backlinks to the respective source article at the end of each guide in Plain Language, in the text section "Where can you get more information?".

4 Prominently placed, but invisible for Google – a dilemma

The described location and anchoring of the translations within the site structure aims at a high accessibility. Users should be able to discover them as easily as possible, navigate through them, and obtain information on health-related topics in Plain Language. To do this, however, they first have to find the page.

Here, we are faced with a problem: the Plain Language guides cannot be found (directly) via a Google search (StatCount 2021, November).[7] Only the landing page (https://www.apotheken-umschau.de/einfache-sprache/) is listed in the search index. This is because we instructed the search engines not to include any of the other texts in Plain Language in the search index (SISTRIX 2021, February 02), in order to avoid a negative impact on the findability of our original texts. By linking the original text and translation so closely, we are creating duplicate content from the search engines' point of view. Google, for example, considers duplicate content as not providing users with any added value. In the search results (SERPs), content identified as duplicate therefore receives a lower ranking. It is thus displayed further down or no longer on the first page of Google search results (cf. ibid.: 2021, August 12). Since our advertising revenue from marketing through the website is strongly linked to its reach and its performance on Google, we cannot afford any fluctuations or drops here.

7 Google stands here pars pro toto for all search engines. With a market share of around 85 % in the past five years, Google is by far the largest provider.

This results in a dilemma that we have not yet been able to solve. Roughly 95 % of visitors to our website come to us via search engines. Compared to the rest of the content on our site, the texts in Plain Language are hardly called up at all and only achieved around 0.1 % of the website's total page impressions (PI) between April and October 2021. For the entire Plain Language offering, that is still about 26,000 page impressions per month (Wort & Bild Verlag 2021), but this seems hardly satisfactory. One possible solution to this dilemma would be to present the Plain Language texts to the search engines as what they are: translations into another language. However, the conditions for this are not currently in place.[8]

The challenge for us now is to actively draw users' attention to our service independently of Google. We do this, for example, by regularly featuring newly published articles in Plain Language in the twice-weekly Apotheken Umschau newsletter (around 58,000 subscribers), posting them on the Apotheken Umschau Facebook channel (https://www.facebook.com/Apotheken.Umschau/; near 180,000 likes and over 185,000 follows) (Wort & Bild Verlag 2021), or referring to our service in press releases on suitable occasions – for example, on International Easy Language Day (Lehmann/Neff-Neudert 2021).

We also use informal exchanges (at trade fairs, congresses or similar occasions) with people working for health institutions, with journalists or business partners to draw attention to our PL services. Another way of creating awareness was through applications for various inclusion or media-related awards. In this way, we hoped to draw the attention of other media professionals and those working in the field of social inclusion to the pioneering work that our service represents in (private-sector) health journalism. One result of these efforts was the award of the Comenius EduMedia Seal for outstanding digital educational media in 2020. With this award, the Society for Pedagogy, Information and Me-

8 It is possible to signal Google to display websites in the appropriate national language or appropriate regional URL. However, this is related to geographical localization and cannot be easily transferred to accessible languages like Easy or Plain Language. In addition, Plain Language and Easy Language would have to be standardized for the respective national language (in our case German) and be able to be specified in ISO 639-1 format. To my knowledge, this standardization does not yet exist. In terms of accessible web services, however, efforts in this direction could be worthwhile (cf. SISTRIX n.d.).

dia "John Amos Comenius" (GPI), "a scientific society for educational media, multimedia, educational technology and mediadidactics [...] honours digital educational media of outstanding content and creative implementation" (GPI 2020). We used this recognition as an opportunity for yet another press release to draw attention to our service (Presseportal 2020, September 25). In addition, we placed the Comenius EduMedia Seal as a quality badge prominently on the landing page of the texts in Plain Language, and – during the first months – even in the header of the entire website.

5 The pandemic, breaking news and Plain Language

While we have not yet found a satisfactory solution to the Google visibility problem, we have been able to effectively and successfully tackle another one: the Covid-19 pandemic was certainly 2020's biggest challenge on a global scale.

As a publisher in the health sector, the onset of the pandemic mid-March 2020[9] forced us to radically change the way we work in the online sector. Previously, we had successfully played the niche of health guides as a special interest medium with our lexical content. Suddenly, we had to compete with virtually all news media in daily news coverage. Responding to this meant a tremendous effort for the entire editorial team. In order to survive in this competition, we first had to create the necessary structures in the organization of our work processes.

Following the protests of various associations of people with disabilities, we realized that for a very long time people with communication impairments had hardly any access to the information about the new coronavirus and the debate around it. Here, we believed we could make a real contribution with our PL service, enabling these people to inform themselves independently and implement the hygiene measures accordingly. On March 25th, 2020, we therefore

9 On January 27, 2020, the first Corona case was confirmed in Germany. On march 11, 2020, the WHO declares the disease a worldwide pandemic. On march 16, 2020, the first lockdown begins in the state of Bavaria. On march 22, 2020, the comprehensive contact restrictions also come into force nationwide. The entire country is now in lockdown (cf. Kunkel 2021, January 27; Bundesregierung 2020, March 22).

published the first guides on Covid-19 in Plain Language (Apotheken Umschau 2021, April 21).[10] Especially at the beginning of the pandemic, it was difficult to stay up to date with our translations. This was because the scientific findings and the official rules of conduct were changing at a fast pace, sometimes on a daily basis. Fortunately, the team of translators at the Research Centre for Easy Language was able to respond very quickly to the constant requests for updates. Thus, we were at least able to keep the core guides on Covid-19 in Plain Language reasonably up-to-date. However, the additional proofreading loop due to the double technical review (linguistic and medical) slowed down the publication process significantly. The PL articles always appeared a few days after the original texts. By then, the research situation had sometimes changed again. Therefore, texts such as the articles on the current measures of the federal government or on hand hygiene had to undergo a second cycle of updating and revision before they could be published at all. But that is a price we had to pay in order to live up to our standards and the Apotheken Umschau brand's promise of providing scientifically sound and tested health information in an easy-to-understand form, even during the pandemic.

Germany's federal structure resulted in a much-lamented patchwork of constantly changing anti-pandemic regulations and measures that differed from state to state. Because of the confusing situation, we focused on making accessible and accurate basic information on the pandemic and the novel coronavirus available to our readers as an absolute priority. Our focus was not on the most recent changes in legal regulations, but primarily on useful information that would guide action. The empirical findings of our partners at the Research Centre for Easy Language on the lifeworld of our target group helped us a great deal in selecting and prioritizing the texts to be translated.

Even though the pandemic situation remained tense for the entire year and the following year of 2021, knowledge about the new coronavirus did not change as rapidly and fundamentally from the second half of 2020 as it did during the first weeks and months of the pandemic, when relatively little was

10 We have since removed some other articles that were published along with this article from the web or incorporated them into other guides. Currently (as of November 2021), we offer nine articles on key topics related to the corona virus in Plain Language.

known about the virus. For the Plain Language texts on Covid-19, this meant that we no longer needed to update them as frequently. New scientific findings on the topic were seldomly so fundamental that we needed to take them into account in the less detailed Plain Language version of the respective texts. We now no longer had texts on the ever-changing political anti-pandemic measures translated. We felt that this information was already sufficiently accessible at the time. Instead, we focused more on our core business of health guides again. From June 2020, we therefore returned to having more of our regular health guides translated into Plain Language. The texts on coronavirus remained prominently placed on the landing page above the other Plain Language guides. However, they have now become part of our regular range of offers.

6 Conclusion: From test run to fully integrated service

In November 2021, a good two years after the test run with the first ten texts in Plain Language went online on 23 September 2019, these translations have evolved into a fully integrated service within the website. https://www.apotheken-umschau.de/einfache-sprache now features more than 150 articles in Plain Language on all kinds of health-related topics. The offer is constantly being expanded and updated as needed. Our aim is to translate the most important topics concerning diseases, medicines and preventive healthcare into Plain Language step by step on our website and to present them in such a way that as many readers as possible can comprehend and benefit from them. We provide this service free of charge and without advertising, and do not make its success dependent on its reach or on its click numbers. We see it as our social responsibility to offer such services as texts in Plain Language. Or as Dennis Ballwieser, Managing Director of Wort & Bild Verlag and Editor-in-Chief of Apotheken Umschau, puts it: "While public authorities and non-profit institutions are obliged to publish texts in Plain Language, this does not yet apply to the free market. But that is not the self-conception of the Apotheken Umschau: It wants to be close to the people. We do this because it is right and important, because we want to, not because we have to" (Apotheken Umschau 2021, May 28).

Literature

Apotheken Umschau (n.d.). Retrieved: 2021, November 22. In: https://www.apotheken-umschau.de/.

Apotheken Umschau (2017, August 30): "Altersbedingte Makuladegeneration (AMD) – Überblick". In: https://www.apotheken-umschau.de/krankheiten-symptome/augenkrankheiten/altersbedingte-makuladegeneration-amd-ueberblick-733645.html, Retrieved: November 30, 2021.

Apotheken Umschau (2019, July 08): "Kurzsichtigkeit: Ursachen und Therapie". In: https://www.apotheken-umschau.de/krankheiten-symptome/augenkrankheiten/kurzsichtigkeit-ursachen-und-therapie-733871.html, Retrieved: November 30, 2021.

Apotheken Umschau (2019, September 23a): "Herzinfarkt". In: https://www.apotheken-umschau.de/einfache-sprache/herzinfarkt-722047.html, Retrieved: November 30, 2021.

Apotheken Umschau (2019, September 23b): "Schlaganfall". In: https://www.apotheken-umschau.de/einfache-sprache/schlaganfall-722079.html, Retrieved: November 30, 2021.

Apotheken Umschau (2019, September 29): "Schlaganfall". In: https://www.apotheken-umschau.de/einfache-sprache/schlaganfall-722079.html, Retrieved: November 30, 2021.

Apotheken Umschau (2020, January 27): "Darmspiegelung". In: https://www.apotheken-umschau.de/einfache-sprache/darmspiegelung-722805.html, Retrieved: November 30, 2021.

Apotheken Umschau (2020, February 06): "Blutvergiftung". In: https://www.apotheken-umschau.de/einfache-sprache/blutvergiftung-723243.html, Retrieved: November 30, 2021.

Apotheken Umschau (2021, March 03): "Altersbedingte Makula-Degeneration". In: https://www.apotheken-umschau.de/einfache-sprache/altersbedingte-makula-degeneration-769785.html, Retrieved: November 30, 2021.

Apotheken Umschau (2021, May 28): "Unser Angebot in 'Einfacher Sprache'". In: https://www.apotheken-umschau.de/krankheiten-symptome/infektionskrankheiten/coronavirus/unser-angebot-in-einfacher-sprache-781547.html, Retrieved: November 15, 2021.

Apotheken Umschau (2021, April 21): "Corona-Virus". In: https://www.apotheken-umschau.de/einfache-sprache/corona-virus-723743.html, Retrieved: November 17, 2021.

Bredel, Ursula/Maaß, Christiane (2016): *Leichte Sprache. Theoretische Grundlagen, Orientierung für die Praxis*. Berlin: Dudenverlag (Sprache im Blick – Duden).

Bundesregierung (2020, March 22): "Besprechung der Bundeskanzlerin mit den Regierungsschefininnen und Regierungschefs der Länder vom 22.03.2020". In: https://www.bundesregierung.de/resource/blob/975226/1733246/e6d6ae0e89a7ffea1ebf6f32cf472736/2020-03-22-mpk-data.pdf?download=1, Retrieved: November 17, 2021.

Gesellschaft für Pädagogik, Information und Medien e. V. (GPI) (2020): "Comenius Award 2020. Call for submissions." In: https://comenius-award.de/wp-content/uploads/2020/09/Comenius_2020_webflyer_EN_V4-03.04.20.pdf, Retrieved: November 28, 2021.

Kunkel, Ulrike (2021, January 27): "Wie das Virus zu uns kam. Ein Jahr Corona in Deutschland". In: https://www.zdf.de/nachrichten/panorama/corona-bayern-china-webasto-100.html, Retrieved: November 17, 2021.

Lehmann, Kai/Neff-Neudert, Katharina (2021): "Unser Angebot in 'Einfacher Sprache'". In: https://www.apotheken-umschau.de/krankheiten-symptome/infektionskrankheiten/coronavirus/unser-angebot-in-einfacher-sprache-781547.html, Retrieved: November 15, 2021.

Maaß, Christiane (2020): *Easy Language – Plain Language – Easy Language Plus. Balancing Comprehensibility and Acceptability*. Berlin: Frank & Timme (Easy – Plain – Accessible; 3), 233–238. <https://library.oapen.org/handle/20.500.12657/42089> Retrieved: November 30, 2021.

Presseportal (2019, October 3019): "apotheken-umschau.de bietet als erstes deutschsprachiges Gesundheitsportal Inhalte in Einfacher Sprache". In: https://www.presseportal.de/pm/52139/4418383, Retrieved: November 29, 2021.

Presseportal (2020, September 25): "Comenius-EduMedia-Award 2020: Auszeichnung für apotheken-umschau.de mit dem Siegel des europäischen Bildungsmedienpreises". In: https://www.presseportal.de/pm/52139/4716744, Retrieved: November 30, 2021.

Schaeffer, Doris et al. (2016): *Gesundheitskompetenz der Bevölkerung in Deutschland: Ergebnisbericht.* Universität Bielefeld. <https://pub.uni-bielefeld.de/download/2908111/2908198/Ergebnisbericht_HLS-GER.pdf> Retrieved: November 30, 2021.

Schaeffer, Doris/Hurrelmann, Klaus/Bauer, Ulrich/Kolpatzik, Kai (eds.) (2018): *National Action Plan Health Literacy. Promoting Health Literacy in Germany*. Berlin: KomPart. <http://www.hlca-consortium.de/wp-content/uploads/2018/06/National-Action-Plan-Health-Literacy.pdf> Retrieved: November 30, 2021.

Schaeffer, Doris/Berens, Eva-Maria/Gille, Svea/Griese, Lennert/Klinger, Julia/de Sombre, Steffen/Vogt, Dominique/Hurrelmann, Klaus (2021): *Gesundheitskompetenz der Bevölkerung in Deutschland – vor und während der Corona Pandemie: Ergebnisse des HLS-GER 2.* Bielefeld: Interdisziplinäres Zentrum für Gesundheitskompetenzforschung (IZGK), Universität Bielefeld. DOI: https://doi.org/10.4119/unibi/2950305.

SISTRIX (n.d.): "The hreflang-guide to international SEO". In: https://www.sistrix.com/hreflang-guide/, Retrieved: November 15, 2021.

SISTRIX (2021, February 02): "Was ist die noindex Anweisung?". In: https://www.sistrix.de/frag-sistrix/robots-noindex/, Retrieved: November 14, 2021.

SISTRIX (2021, August 12): "Duplicate Content". In: https://www.sistrix.de/frag-sistrix/onpage/duplicate-content/, Retrieved: November 14, 2021.

StatCounter (2021, November): "Marktanteile der meistgenutzten Suchmaschinen auf dem Desktop nach Page Views weltweit von Januar 2016 bis Oktober 2021". In: https://de.statista.com/statistik/daten/studie/225953/umfrage/die-weltweit-meistgenutzten-suchmaschinen/, Retrieved: November 14, 2021.

Wort & Bild Verlag (2021): "Einfache Sprache auf apotheken-umschau.de. Ad hoc-Reporting, 23.11.2021". In: file:///Users/julian.hoerner/Downloads/Einfache%20Sprache_auswertung_2021-11-23.pdf,Retrieved: November 28, 2021. Unpublished.

Loraine Keller

Digital Participation or Digital Divide?

The role of the media barrier, acceptance and trust in health information from the perspective of elderly users

1 Introduction

Especially in old age, the need for health information grows with the increase of (chronic) diseases (cf. RKI 2014). The most common reason to seek health information is having acute symptoms of illness oneself or looking for information for someone close who is affected (Baumann/Link 2020: 682). One of the fastest possibilities to get health information nowadays is via internet, which offers countless pages of content. One problem when using online offers to seek health information is having to figure out whether a page contains serious information or if the quality of the content just pursues economic (or other) interests (Koch 2017: 57; e.g., clickbaiting). People with low health literacy find it especially hard to appraise (online) health information (Schaeffer et al. 2021: 68). In Germany, 86 % of people aged 65 and over have problematic (7.3 %) or inadequate digital health literacy (78.7 %) (ibid.). They use digital information options the least: Although over 40 % of them use internet sites on the topic of health, they are also the group with the lowest use of all age groups considered in the second Health Literacy Survey in Germany (ibid.). This article will focus on the question of whether people, in particular the elderly, actually use online content and what could be reasons for the non-use of digital health information offers.

2 Media barrier and trust

Rink (2020) identifies several types of barriers that can hinder the reception process on the user or the text side. The media barrier can refer to the areas of codality, modality and the medium itself (Rink 2019: 32). Codality is concerned when a particular sign system in which linguistic information is encoded cannot be decoded (ibid.). A barrier with regard to modality is present when the sensory organ that is needed to perceive the information is not functional (ibid.). The medium itself can also become a barrier, namely when it is not accessible (enough) to the recipients as a carrier of information (ibid., cf. Rink 2020). This is the case when a certain group of recipients does not have access to entire media contents because they rarely or never use the medium, as is the case, for example, with many older people when it comes to contents from the internet (Rink 2019: 59). The specific needs and forms of use determine the preferred access of these people to content through certain media (ibid. 32; for the specific needs and preferences of elderly recipients see Keller in prep.; cf. chapters below).

Trust is inherent to media preference(s) and consists of the positive expectations someone has towards a certain content, person etc. (cf. Link 2019: 51). In the following chapters, the relation of trust and acceptance with regard to *media access*, *competences* and *preferences* will be explained to show how the media barrier can potentially be overcome for elderly seekers of health information. The interdependence between media access, preferences and competences and potential barriers on the way to successful retrieval of information for this target group is modelled after the first findings of a current study (Keller in prep.).

2.1 Media access

As proposed in the opening article of this volume , the first step in the Hildesheim school's accessible communication model is to be able to retrieve information (cf. Maaß/Rink 2019; Maaß 2020). If recipients cannot retrieve information or the retrieval requires too much capacity, the comprehension process can be terminated before the information is processed (see introductory article in this volume). Reasons for the non-retrievability of online information on the user side can be found in the digital divide: There are differences in access as well as in skills and uses of information and communication technologies that are linked to social inequalities (Hargittai/Hsieh 2013: 130–137). On the first-level digital divide, differences in access can be found at an individual as well as on a nation-state level (ibid. 132). This can be the case if there is no internet connection, e.g. in rural areas, or if there are no mobile devices available with which to go online. This is often due to a lower socioeconomic status (Hargittai/Hsieh 2013: 131). In these cases, people would potentially be able to navigate and use online content, if access was granted or affordable.

The question of whether social class differences are turning into digital class differences is not new (Hargittai 2002; Bonfadelli 2019). Digitalization must not reinforce class, education and income differences, but reduce them (cf. Hargittai/Hsieh 2013: 141–42). This requires an education programme that includes everyone. Rifts of digital divide run through the entire population; even within the group of older people, there are large differences in media competence with digital media or technological equipment, depending on the level of education (cf. Bonfadelli 2019: 353). Access should be made easier, e.g. through uniform user interfaces for the various digital media, so that ever-increasing innovations do not deny access again: As the Eighth Ageing Report of the Federal Government in Germany puts it with regard to social integration, attention must be "drawn to the danger of exacerbating social inequalities, because people with better education and greater income resources can make better use of digital opportunities than people with fewer resources. The latter, in particular, run the risk of losing social contacts in the increasingly digitalised world. It is important to counteract this by making special offers available for this target group" (BMFSFJ 2020: 12; own translation).

Older people should not be seen as passive, but should be explicitly involved in identifying themselves with central digital products and also in implementing the technologies (cf. ibid.). Furthermore, an education programme is necessary so that potential users can be taught and accompanied in the use of digital technologies (see next chapter).

Digitalization is particularly important in questions of participation, e.g., exchange with others or ordering services, e.g., also of medicines, especially when people in old age are more and more bound to their homes, which became particularly apparent in the COVID-19 pandemic in 2020 (cf. Kruse 2020). Digitalization holds a lot of opportunities if access to digital offers is granted. Access includes availability of Wi-Fi and devices, which are especially inadequate in facilities for the elderly or internet connections and speed in rural areas (cf. BMFSFJ 2020: 38).

2.2 Media Competences

On the second-level digital divide, the reasons for non-use lie in the lack of user competence with the medium: Recipients are not able to use devices, to find their way around the internet itself or to navigate web pages. As in the first-level digital divide, this is strongly linked to the factors of education level and income, as well as age (cf. Hargittai/Hsieh 2013: 135). Especially elderly people who did not grow up with the medium internet are often not used to navigating the internet or to operating the devices necessary to go online (cf. Stiel 2021). The low level of competence with digital technologies among older people is mainly due to a lack of opportunities for experience, especially if they did not experience digital technologies e.g. at work or elsewhere (ibid.). With regard to neuronal plasticity, gerontologists state that it is present in older people: Lifelong learning and development is possible even in old age, but the competences and the ability to learn must then be supported, if necessary, by assisting persons in dealing with and operating digital media (BMFSFJ 2020: 58, Croll 2020). The ability to learn depends on biographical characteristics; according to the gerontologist Andreas Kruse (2020), the neurologic ability to learn does not decline in old age. Studies that question the learning ability of older people must be carefully evaluated: If the level of abstraction of the tasks or the subject in question is adapted to the biography of the older participants, this is also reflected in the results. An educated person will achieve better results than a less educated one, those who like to learn will possibly be better at handling the respective digital medium more quickly, etc. (Kruse 2020). Next to cognitive abilities, computer anxiety can also contribute to the negative relationship between (old) age and information and communication technologies (Czaja et al. 2006, cf. Hargittai/Hsieh 2013: 134–135). To avoid a motivational barrier even before the retrieval of information (cf. Lang 2021), it is crucial to introduce elderly users to digital technologies, to practice navigation and orientation and thus reduce negative feelings or anxieties towards internet use.

From 2015 to 2020, the German "KommmiT" (Communication with Intelligent Technology) project developed and tested measures "to introduce people who are inexperienced in technology and have limited mobility to the digital world in a targeted manner and to strengthen the networking of these people" (LFK 2020: KommmiT, own translation). Nine partners from the fields of science, industry, geriatric care and the public sector developed a holistic concept to enable older, technology-inexperienced people to gain digital access and furthermore, social and digital participation (ibid.).

Efforts such as the "KommmiT" project in Stuttgart or the "Digitaler Engel" (in English "Digital Angel", a bus touring Germany to teach older people about the use of digital offers on a day-to-day basis,) support elderly people personally and locally in concrete questions of digital offers (cf. Digitaler Engel (n.d.).): Über das Projekt). Furthermore, there are guides for introducing senior citizens to digital offerings, such as the guide by the Digital Opportunities Foundation in cooperation with Telefonica Deutschland, which contains a brief overview of individual topics as well as a glossary with relevant explanations of terms such as USB, Bluetooth or Cloud (see Stiftung Digitale Chancen (Digital Opportunities Foundation) 2019: Leitfaden). These efforts can help to reduce the fear of digital technology usage for elderly people and enable them to integrate new sources of information and communication in their everyday lives.

2.3 Media preferences

Another reason that is strongly neglected in most cases is the media preference of users: If potential users do not choose to use the medium internet via any possible device, the information, as comprehensible and action-oriented as it may be, will not be found (cf. Maaß 2020). Closely linked to the media preference is the concept of trust in different media or media content: Trust is inherent to media preference(s) and consists, not only in the context of media preferences, of the positive expectations someone has towards a certain content, person etc. (cf. Link 2019: 51). Trust serves the trusting individual as a means to overcome insecurities (ibid.). In terms of media preferences, this means that a person chooses to use his/her favourite media in most of the cases and that he or she is willing to give their favourite medium or the content offered the benefit of the doubt. This may be the case because it has fulfilled their needs in most of the cases, e.g. to find a satisfying answer to an urgent health question or to get a hint regarding other sources of information or contacts (for the relation between acceptance, satisfaction and continuous usage intention see Momani 2018). Sometimes, the features of a medium make it attractive to users and thus lead to a certain preference (e.g. TV as a preferred medium for recipients with reading difficulties or who do not like reading; Keller in prep.). Trust in the given information is often linked to the person (e.g. health experts such as doctors, physiotherapists etc.) or institution that is associated with the information, no matter whether these are really responsible for the given content:

In Germany, pharmacies offer issues of the magazine "Apotheken Umschau" which can be picked up in local pharmacies or can be delivered directly to a household along with ordered medicine. In a recent study (Keller in prep.), older people often state that they pick up different issues at their pharmacies or get them delivered, e.g. the special issue for senior citizens (Seniorenratgeber) or for diabetics (Diabetesratgeber). These issues are then evaluated as very trustworthy because they come from their local pharmacies and are estimated to be written by experts "who are experienced and foremost doctors" (cf. Keller in prep.). The participants even defend the magazine in terms of the included advertisements which "do not have to do anything with the articles" (cf. Keller in prep.). They also highlight that these issues of the magazine are for free which is an important factor for their reception (cf. Braun 2017: 55). Accessibility – also in a financial sense – is crucial when it comes to user preferences of health information. Also, the participants prefer these print versions of health information to online information and appreciate the fact that there are issues which are particularly tailored to their needs as senior citizens or to special health conditions such as diabetes. In order to create positive social distinctiveness and to valorise their own (age) group, people choose media formats in which their own age group (or other group forms, for example supporters of a certain political party) is positively evaluated (cf. Trepte & Loy 2017, Trepte et al. 2021: 71).

As stated, trust is inherent in the participants' media preferences. A media barrier can occur in the users' preferences, competences and/or access to different media and hinder the process of reception right at the first step of retrieving the information (Maaß 2020; Maaß/Rink 2019).

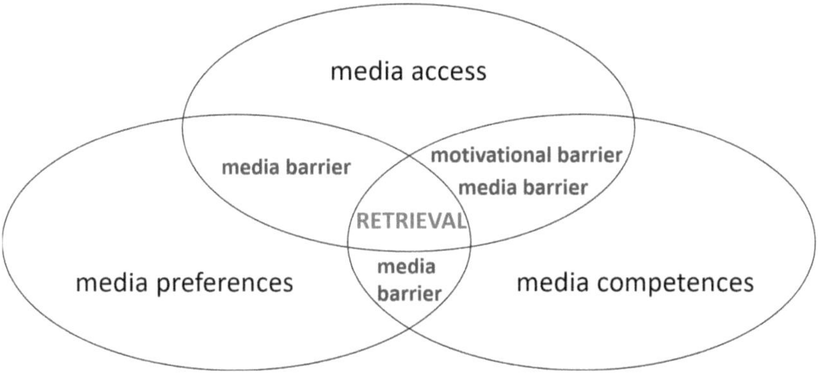

Figure 1: The interdependence between media access, preferences and competences and potential barriers on the way to successful retrieval of information (Keller in prep.)

The illustration shows the relation and interdependence between access, preferences and competences with regard to media content. The former can only be successfully retrieved, if access is granted and the user's preferences and competences match the medium that is offering the content. Only if the recipients' preferences and competences overlap with the possibility of access (which can depend more than the former two aspects on exterior factors like the socio-technological setting in the potential usage situation, see section *Media Access*), the media barrier (and, in case of different media preferences, the motivational barrier) will not hinder the reception process. If for one of the three aspects a media (or motivational) barrier occurs, the successful retrieval as the first step of the accessible communication process (cf. Maaß 2020; Maaß/Rink 2019), cannot take place. Then, the following steps of perception, comprehension, recall and especially of acceptance of the communication offer will not be successfully passed and thus the user will not be able to act on the given information (cf. ibid.).

3 Acceptance is key

Trust goes hand in hand with acceptance (cf. Link 2019: 88). Acceptance is crucial at every step of the reception process and can be hindered by the media barrier (Rink 2020, Maaß 2020), especially if target groups who are hard to reach are at the centre of the content (cf. Reifegerste 2014): These are elderly people, people with low income and education or people who have obstructing conditions that go together with the known factors, enhancing the digital divide, such as living in rural areas, having a migration background and, as already mentioned, having a low socioeconomic status (ibid.; cf. Hargittai/Hsieh 2013). These hard-to-reach groups match the groups identified as having a (very) low health literacy in Germany (Schaeffer et al. 2018).

Acceptance is a social phenomenon that can be found "across different spheres of rationalisation and areas of life in all social groupings (e.g. status groups)" (Lang 2017: 20). Acceptance can thus be understood as a fundamental feature of action and structure of interpersonal coexistence (ibid.). With regard to the choice of media, it is primarily a matter of attitudinal psychological access to acceptance (cf. ibid.): Acceptance is the *willingness* to accept a medium, person, etc. Acceptance is visible in the practical consequences and concrete results of action (ibid. 23), such as the choice of a certain medium. Statistics on media use show that the average use of the internet by older people is much lower than it is in other age groups (Destatis 2021, Bonfadelli 2019: 353). In their *Unified Theory of Acceptance and Use of Technology*, Venkatesh et al. (2003) name age as one of the factors that can have an influence on the determinants of usage intention und actual usage behaviour. Further factors are gender, experience and the voluntariness of use (ibid.). Determinants of usage intention are performance expectancy, effort expectancy, social influence, while the fourth determinant, facilitating conditions, is directly linked to user behaviour (ibid.).

To ensure the acceptance of health information, providers have to consider the media preferences, the needs and conditions of the everyday life of their target group. The central feature of a person's identity is their lifestyle. The continuity of everyday life is important so that a person can feel comfortable within it and can control and shape it (Kruse 2020; BMFSFJ 2020). For younger people, their own lifeworld is already strongly determined by digital technology (Dutton et al. 2009, Hargittai/Hsieh 2013). For older people, digital technologies should be understood as an offer that they *can* use, but *do not have to* (Kruse 2020). Providers need to take a close look at the *willingness* – as Venkatesh et al. (2003) put it, the usage intention – of their recipients to use certain media and take into account the various reasons due to which a preference or non-use can occur. In a recent study (Keller in prep.), the factors for the occurrence of a media barrier at the first step of the reception process, the retrieval of information, and thus for the use or non-use of the medium internet by the participants are linked as follows:

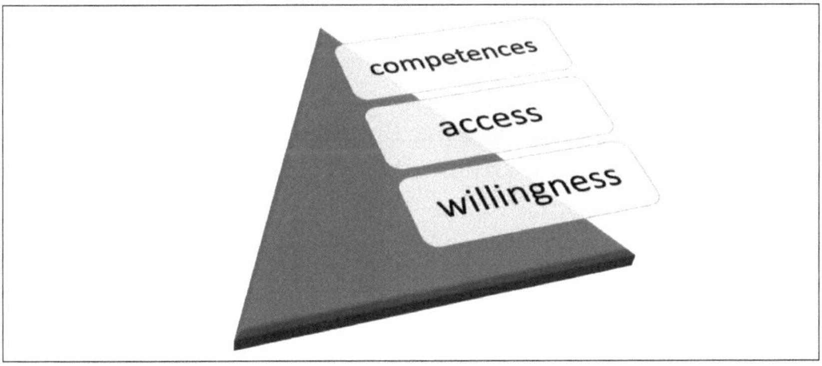

Figure 2: The steps to online health information usage for elderly users (Keller in prep.)

If the recipient is willing to use the internet, it is the first step towards usage. Willingness comprises the preferences and motivation of the user: If he or she does not like going online, the usage will be denied by this preference, even if the access and competence(s) for it are given. If, however, the user is willing to use the internet, the next step, access, can be taken. If access is also granted, if there is a connection and a device to go online with, the next step can be taken: The recipient has to be competent enough to use the medium, navigate it and retrieve the searched information. If all of these steps have been successfully taken, actual usage of online (health) information will occur[1]. Otherwise, content creators – not only in the field of health information – have to think about other ways to reach the intended audience.

4 Conclusion

In Germany, as in other societies in Western countries, the population has grown older much faster in the last decades (cf. Destatis 2019). As elderly people in particular are in need of health information due to the fact that health problems increase even more with age, the need to focus on adequate health information for this target group becomes inevitable (cf. Maaß 2020). This group often falls behind when it comes to the use of the internet as a quick and direct information source. Not only the access via connection and devices needs to be given for the recipients to actually use the internet, but also the competences and the willingness on the users' side. As shown above, the interdependence between media access, preferences and competences and potential barriers has to be considered on the way to successful retrieval of online health information. As elderly people often prefer classic media such as TV or (print) newspaper to seek health information and put a lot of trust in them (cf. Keller in prep.), health information providers need to take into account these preferences in order to reach the intended audience. As for the equipment necessary for access and in terms of gaining individual competences in internet use, political action has to be taken to enable elderly people who will be otherwise left out not only digitally, but also socially.

1 This illustration focuses on the first step in the reception process: Online information can be actually retrieved and the media barrier can be overcome at this point of the process. Other barrier types (cf. Rink 2020) linked to the following steps of the reception process can occur later, e.g. if the information comprises too much expert language etc. (see introduction of this vol.).

Literature

Bonfadelli, Heinz (2019): "Wissenskluft-Perspektive und Digital Divide in der Gesundheitskommunikation." In: Rossmann, Constanze/Hastall, Matthias R. (eds.): *Handbuch der Gesundheitskommunikation*. Wiesbaden: Springer, pp. 347–357.

Braun, Bernard (2017): "Patentrezept Medienkompetenz. Ein Weg zur Steigerung der Gesundheitskompetenz?". In: *Public Health Forum* 2017; 25 (1), pp. 54–56.

Bundesministerium für Familie, Senioren, Frauen und Jugend (BMFSFJ) (2020): *Achter Bericht zur Lage der älteren Generation in der Bundesrepublik Deutschland. Ältere Menschen und Digitalisierung*. Drucksache 19/21650. Berlin: BMFSFJ.

Croll, Jutta (2020): *Empfehlungen des Achten Altersberichts weiterdenken*. Vortrag auf der Online-Konferenz "Leben im Alter unter Pandemie-Bedingungen: Digitalisierung als Chance" am 19.11.2020 der Landesinitiative Niedersachsen Generationengerechter Alltag (LINGA) in Kooperation mit der Landesvereinigung für Gesundheit und Akademie für Sozialmedizin Niedersachsen e.V.

Czaja, Sara J./Charness, Neil/Fisk, Arthur D./Hertzog, Christopher/Nair, Sankaran N./Rogers, Wendy A./Sharit, Joseph (2006): "Factors predicting the use of technology: findings from the Center for Research and Education on Aging and Technology Enhancement (CREATE)". In: *Psychol Aging*. 21 (2), pp. 333–352.

Destatis (2021): *Internetnutzung von Personen 2020*. Statistisches Bundesamt (Destatis). https://www.destatis.de/DE/Themen/Gesellschaft-Umwelt/Einkommen-Konsum-Lebensbedingungen/_Grafik/_Interaktiv/it-nutzung-alter.html (last access 22.11.2021).

Destatis (2019): "*Bevölkerung im Wandel: Ergebnisse der 14. Koordinierten Bevölkerungsvorausberechnung*" am 27. Juni 2019 in Berlin, Statement. Wiesbaden: Statistisches Bundesamt (Destatis).

Digitaler Engel (o.J.): *Über das Projekt*. https://www.digitaler-engel.org/ (19.11.2020).

Dutton, William H./Helsper, Ellen J./Gerber, Monica M. (2009): *The Internet in Britain: 2009*. Oxford Internet Institute, University of Oxford.

Hargittai, Eszter (2002): "Second-Level Digital Divide: Differences in People's Online Skills". In: *First Monday* 7 (4).

HARGITTAI, ESZTER/HSIEH, YULI PATRICK (2013): "Digital Inequality". In: DUTTON, WILLIAM H. (eds.): *The Oxford Handbook of Internet Studies*. Oxford: University Press, pp. 129–150.

KELLER, LORAINE (i. prep.): *Verständlichkeitsoptimierte Medizinkommunikation. Akzeptabilität und Akzeptanz von Texten in Einfacher und Leichter Sprache*. Manuskript der Dissertationsschrift. Hildesheim: Universität Hildesheim.

KOCH, KLAUS (2017): "Informationen aus dem Internet". In: *Public Health Forum* 25 (1), pp. 57–59.

KRUSE, ANDREAS (2020): *Ältere Menschen und Digitalisierung. Erkenntnisse und Empfehlungen des Achten Altersberichts der Bundesregierung*. Vortrag auf der Online-Konferenz "Leben im Alter unter Pandemie-Bedingungen: Digitalisierung als Chance" am 19.11.2020 der Landesinitiative Niedersachsen Generationengerechter Alltag (LINGA) in Kooperation mit der Landesvereinigung für Gesundheit und Akademie für Sozialmedizin Niedersachsen e.V.

Landesanstalt für Kommunikation (LFK) (2020): *KommmiT*. https://www.lfk.de/medienkompetenz/seniorinnen-und-senioren/kommmit (19.11.2020).

LANG, GERT (2017): *Zur Akzeptanz sozialer Ungleichheit. Theoretische Überlegungen und empirische Befunde zur gesellschaftlichen Kohärenz*. Wiesbaden: Springer Fachmedien.

LANG, KATRIN (2021): *Auffindbarkeit, Wahrnehmbarkeit, Akzeptabilität. Webseiten von Behörden in Leichter Sprache vor dem Hintergrund der rechtlichen Lage*. Berlin: Frank & Timme.

MAAẞ, CHRISTIANE (2020): *Easy Language – Plain Language – Easy Language Plus. Balancing Comprehensibility and Acceptability*. Berlin: Frank & Timme.

MAAẞ, CHRISTIANE/RINK, ISABEL (2019): "Über das Handbuch Barrierefreie Kommunikation". In: MAAẞ, CHRISTIANE/RINK, ISABEL (eds.): *Handbuch Barrierefreie Kommunikation*. Berlin: Frank & Timme, pp. 17–25.

MOMANI, A. M. (2018). *Adoption of Acceptance Theory and Social Commerce Use (TAUSC Model) for Consumer Behaviour*. Al-Madinah International University.

REIFEGERSTE, DOREEN (2014): "Gesundheitskommunikation für schwer erreichbare Zielgruppen". In: HURRELMANN, KLAUS/BAUMANN, EVA (eds.): *Handbuch Gesundheitskommunikation*. Bern: Verlag Hans Huber, pp. 170–181.

Rink, Isabel (2019): "Kommunikationsbarrieren". In: Maaß, Christiane/Rink, Isabel (eds.): *Handbuch Barrierefreie Kommunikation*. Berlin: Frank & Timme, pp. 29–65.

Rink, Isabel (2020): *Rechtskommunikation und Barrierefreiheit. Zur Übersetzung juristischer Informations- und Interaktionstexte in Leichte Sprache*. Berlin: Frank & Timme.

RKI – Robert Koch-Institut (ed.) (2014): *Chronisches Kranksein. Faktenblatt zu GEDA 2012: Ergebnisse der Studie "Gesundheit in Deutschland aktuell 2012"*. RKI, Berlin.

Schaeffer, Doris/Berens, Eva-Maria/Gille, Svea/Griese, Lennart/Klinger, Julia/de Sombre, Steffen/Vogt, Dominique/Hurrelmann, Klaus (2021): *Gesundheitskompetenz der Bevölkerung in Deutschland – vor und während der Corona Pandemie: Ergebnisse des HLS-GER 2*. Bielefeld: Interdisziplinäres Zentrum für Gesundheitskompetenzforschung (IZGK), Universität Bielefeld.

Schaeffer, Doris/Hurrelmann, Klaus/Bauer, Ullrich/Kolpatzik, Kai (2018): *Nationaler Aktionsplan Gesundheitskompetenz. Die Gesundheitskompetenz in Deutschland stärken*. 1st revised edition. Berlin: KomPart.

Stiel, Janina (2021): *Älteren den Einstieg in die digitale Welt erleichtern* [Bundesarbeitsgemeinschaft der Seniorenorganisationen e.V.]. Presentation at the 10th BZgA regional conference "Gesund und aktiv älter werden [Growing old actively and healthy]" in Schleswig-Holstein. Online conference. July 2021, Landesvereinigung für Gesundheitsförderung in Schleswig-Holstein e.V.

Stiftung Digitale Chancen (2019): *Leitfaden Digitale Kompetenzen für ältere Menschen. So plane und gestalte ich Angebote zur Unterstützung von Senioren*. 2. erweiterte Auflage. Berlin: Stiftung Digitale Chancen.

Trepte, Sabine/Loy, Laura S. (2017): "Social Identity Theory and Self-Categorization Theory". In: Rössler, Patrick/Hoffner, Cynthia/Zoonen, Liesbet van (eds.): *The International Encyclopedia of Media Effects*. John Wiley and Sons, pp. 1832–1845.

Trepte, Sabine/Reinecke, Leonard/Schäwel, Johanna (2021): *Medienpsychologie*. 3rd extended and revised edition. Stuttgart: W. Kohlhammer.

Venkatesh, Viswanath/Morris, Michael G./Davis, Gordon B./Davis, Fred D. (2003): "User Acceptance of Information Technology: Toward a Unified View". In: *Management Information Systems Quarterly*, 27 (3), pp. 425–478.

Janina Kröger / Sarah Ahrens

An interdisciplinary approach to translation-oriented text analysis in intralingual translation research

Research report

1 Introduction

Communication in the health domain can be found in different communication situations, between people of different levels or fields of expertise and through different media. Health communication often takes place between medical experts and non-experts with the aim of exchanging information. Communication can be oral or written, both of which can present barriers to the people involved. Schaeffer et al. (2021) have shown that understanding health information can be difficult for vulnerable groups. In order to improve accessibility of health information, we must first understand which barriers arise in texts; only then can we translate (understood as overcoming communication barriers, see Hansen-Schirra/Maaß 2019). To understand the textual barriers, we need a text analysis schema. In interlingual translation, the New Rhetoric Formula (Nord 1992, 2009) can be used to analyse a standard text in preparation for the translation process, but it is also applicable to text analysis for research purposes. Yet, there is no such schema for research (nor practice) in intralingual translation.

This contribution is part of the theoretical underpinning of two dissertation projects (Kröger in prep.; Ahrens in prep.)[1]. Both projects are situated at the

1 Both projects are funded by the Robert Bosch Stiftung via the interdisciplinary stipend programme Chronic Diseases and Health Literacy ("Chronische Erkrankungen und Gesundheitskompetenz" (ChEG)).

intersection of accessible communication (Deilen/Hansen-Schirra/Maaß 2019) and health literacy, a research field in the field of public health. From this interdisciplinary standpoint, we will report on our text analysis schema, which is based on the accessible communication model (accessible communication) (Maaß/Rink 2019: 24; Hernández Garrido et al. in print), the New Rhetoric Formula (translation studies) (Nord 1992; 2009), and qualitative content analysis (social studies) (Kuckartz 2016; Kuckartz/Rädiker 2022). The latter influenced the use of, among other tools, MaxQDA as a computer-based tool for text analysis.

In Chapter 2 we will describe the accessible communication model, the New Rhetoric Formula, and qualitative content analysis using, among others, the software MaxQDA. Chapter 3 will show how to combine them to achieve a translation-oriented text analysis schema for the identification of communication barriers in two different research projects. Using the example of passive and passive alternatives, we will use the three models and methods to identify the barriers emerging from these two linguistic phenomena and where they emerge in a text. In Chapter 4, we will discuss advantages and disadvantages of applying our proposed analysis schema in research projects.

2 Models and methods

In this chapter we will describe the accessible communication model (Maaß/Rink 2019, Hernández Garrido et al. in print), the New Rhetoric Formula (Nord 1992; 2009) and qualitative content analysis (Kuckartz 2016; Kuckartz/Rädiker 2022). We will emphasise specific computer-based tools that can support the analysis.

2.1 Accessible communication model

Accessible communication is a newly developing research area. Maaß/Rink (2019: 24) proposed an accessible communication model centred around the text and user perspective on accessible information. This model has been refined and extended by recent research projects (Rink 2020; Lang 2021; Hernández Garrido et al. in print; see Ahrens et al. this volume). Accessible texts have certain text qualities: They are retrievable, perceptible, comprehensible, linkable, acceptable, and action-oriented (Maaß 2020; Hernández Garrido in print; see Ahrens et al. this volume). The steps towards accessible communication and their connection to Health Literacy have been examined in Ahrens et al. (this volume). These steps serve as the point of departure for the proposed source text analysis. Each of these qualities is linked to certain text features and can be affected by the communication barriers according to Rink (2019) and Lang (2021; see also Ahrens et al. this volume). For example, comprehensibility is linked to text qualities such as syntax structure and use of expert terminology which can contribute to a (expert) language barrier. To successfully analyse how accessible a text is with regards to these steps and which text features contribute to the barriers, a schema for analysis is necessary (Chapter 3).

2.2 New Rhetoric Formula

In translation studies, the translation scopos guides the source text (ST) analysis and the planning of the target text (TT). For translation-oriented text analysis, different text analysis schemas are available. For our research purposes, we chose Nord's comprehensive, yet easy to use analysis schema *New Rhetoric Formula*. It is equipped for TT analysis, too, and can thus be used to plan the TT and to consider its communication situation, a feature especially relevant in intralingual translation (Rink in prep.).

Nord (1992: 43; 2009) expands the Lasswell formula "Who says what in which channel to whom with what effect?" to her New Rhetoric Formula. Tables 1–3 list the elements that are analysed according to this formula (cf. Nord 1992: 43; Nord 2009: 160). With her New Rhetoric Formula, Nord (1992) presents a formula for source text (ST) analysis as well as translation scopos and target text (TT) planning. It is a formula grounded in translation studies that is applicable to practice and research. In this chapter, we examine Nord's formula for usability in accessible communication and intralingual translation research.

Nord (1992) distinguishes *intratextual factors*[2] from *extratextual factors* and proposes to analyse the *effect on the reader* separately. The latter is based

2 For improved readability, Nord's terminology will appear in cursive.

on both *intra-* and *extratextual factors*, and is situated within the user perspective (see Maaß 2020). It will therefore not be covered in this contribution that is focused on the text perspective. The *extra-* and *intratextual factors* can be interpreted depending on the text and text type.

extratextual factors	**analysed features**
Who transmits	author, sender
to whom	addressee(s)
what for	sender's intention
by which medium	medium
where	place
when	time
why a text	motive for communication
with what function?	function

Table 1: *Extratextual factors* (Nord 1992: 43; Nord 2009: 160)

intratextual factors	**analysed features**
On what subject matter	topic
does he say what	content
(what not)	knowledge presuppositions
in what order	text structure
using which non-verbal elements	non-verbal elements
in which words	lexis
in what kinds of sentences	syntax
in which tone?	tone, suprasegmental features

Table 2: *Intratextual factors* (Nord 1992: 43; Nord 2009: 160)

interplay of extra- and intratextual factors	**analysed features**
To what effect?	effect on the reader(s)

Table 3: Interplay of *extra-* and *intratextual factors* (Nord 1992: 43; Nord 2009: 160)

Extratextual factors (Table 1) are analysed to correctly interpret the text. In terms of transmission of the text, either *sender* or *author* can be more significant, for example concerning the acceptability of the text. In literary text types, the *author* might be more relevant, whereas in health communication, the *sender* (i.e. the distributor) may be more relevant: Is the text sent (i.e. distributed) by an ad-driven journalistic company or by a state-funded health institution?

The *sender's intention* is relevant in judging the reliability of information, especially in health communication (see for example Sun et al. 2019: 11; for a distinction between health information and marketing texts see Deutsches Netzwerk Evidenzbasierte Medizin e. V. 2016) and thus to the acceptability of the ST.

Place and *time* are relevant influences in judging the topicality and relevance of a text. *Place* is related to *medium*, particularly in online communication, but also to how relevant a text is to the *addressees*. Readers are motivated to read a text if they perceive it as relevant (see Grice 1975: 46f.; Lang 2021: 327). Texts about the German health care system are more relevant to readers in Germany than they are to readers in Austria. The *medium* of the ST relates to retrievability as well as acceptability of the texts (see Keller in this volume).

Addressees are one of the most important factors to analyse – especially in intralingual translation. A ST may be addressed to a broad audience of standard readers with a need for or an interest in the ST, while the TT may address people with cognitive impairments in particular. It is relevant to analyse the characteristics of the *addressees* in order to anticipate *knowledge* and other *presuppositions* (see Chapter 3).

The *motive for communication* is an external influence that motivates the communicative act, for example a global pandemic or a recent study on smoking cessation. It is separate from the *sender's intention* which may be to inform or to appeal. The *motive for communication* may influence the *sender's intention*, while the *sender's intention* influences the text *function*.

Table 2 lists the *intratextual factors*. STs are analysed in translation and translation research to review a ST's applicability for a) the target groups and b) the translation process. In intralingual translation, contents must often be reduced to achieve an acceptable text length (Maaß/Rink 2020: 45f.). Therefore, text *topic* and text *contents* are particularly relevant. For intralingual translation, Rink (in prep.) suggests performing the TT analysis first (i.e. analysis of the communication situation and the *addressees*, for example) before the ST analysis. In interlingual translation, Nord's formula is usable for both ST analysis and TT analysis.

In the same vein, *knowledge presuppositions* in the ST must be reviewed. In comprehensibility-enhanced communication, not only *knowledge presuppositions* must be identified, but also *presuppositions* about literacy and numeracy, two core elements of health literacy (see Ahrens et al. in this volume). The factor *knowledge presuppositions* must thus be broadened for intralingual translation. It is advisable to analyse this factor after the other *intralingual factors*: After all explicit information has been analysed, the implicit *knowledge presuppositions* can be detected more easily.

The analysis of the ST *structure* is necessary to identify issues in comprehensibility and action-orientation of a text – especially in texts that are addressed to more than one target group, such as administrative texts (Rink 2020). Administrative texts, which also exist in the health domain, are structured according to administrative processes instead of comprehensibility and action-orientation (Rink 2020).

Non-verbal elements must be analysed in their interaction with the written text. It is important to analyse their function (decorative, informational etc., see Weidenmann 2002), their perceptibility, their comprehensibility, and their acceptability by the respective target group (for the latter see for example Lázaro Gutiérrez 2017).

Lexis and *syntax* can be analysed with respect to their perceptibility and comprehensibility. Relevant function words or morphemes such as negations might be skipped during the reading process, thus inhibiting comprehension. Long compound nouns may be difficult to perceive while reading, because they may be difficult to segment (Inhoff et al. 2000; Lang 2021: 97; Deilen 2020: 241). Long sentences overload working memory capacity, making comprehension difficult (see Bredel/Maaß 2016: 129).

Tone must be analysed to identify emotion and motivation barriers that affect the acceptability of a text. For this factor, direct and indirect reader-address may be analysed, but also word choices that restrict a reader's personal choice (Rink 2020) like the modal verb "must" (see Chapter 3.1).

It is evident that Nord's formula can be used for accessibility-oriented text analysis with only minor changes, such as a broadened understanding of *knowledge presuppositions* and the enhanced relevance of the *addressees* (see Chapters 3.3 und 4). The relation between the qualities of accessible texts, the communication barriers (see Chapter 2.1), and the New Rhetoric Formular have been described. In further research, and in specific study designs, the relation can be examined in more detail. For this contribution, we focus on Nord's *intratextual factors* (see Chapter 3). In the following chapter, Kuckartz' (2016) qualitative content analysis will be presented.

2.3 Software-aided text analysis

There are several different computer-based tools that can enrich the research-focussed, accessibility-oriented text analysis. Each of the tools presented here has a different focus and thus introduces different aspects into the analysis. At the core of this chapter is the software MaxQDA (Verbi 2022) and how researchers can use it to analyse a text. MaxQDA is software to analyse qualitative data and offers several useful tools (see Chapter 3.3). At the centre of content analyses[3] with MaxQDA are codes, which are derived from classification of items (Kuckartz 2016: 31). The codes are both a tool for analysis and "the substance of the research and the building blocks of the theory the researchers want to develop" (Kuckartz 2019: 183). Similar text features with regards to the research question are collected within a code.

Codes can be developed in three ways: deductively, inductively, and by mixing a deductive and inductive approach (ibid.)[4]. Developing codes deductively means using existing theories, literature, and the research question

3 The method used in MaxQDA is taken from qualitative content analysis as proposed by Kuckartz (2016). Qualitative content analysis is a method to analyse qualitative data, e.g. interviews, tweets or videos, used in social studies as well as in public health. We will show that this method can also be used for text analysis in the context of intralingual translation.

4 Kuckartz prefers the terms concept-driven and data-driven, as the terms inductive and deductive refer to logical consequences of premises or data whereas "the formation of categories based on the state of research, a theory or an advanced hypothesis is very different" (2019: 185). He concedes that the pair inductive – deductive is used in the formation of codes as well (ibid.).

to define codes before analysing the material (ibid.), e.g. features of expert language as defined by literature. Using an inductive approach means using a "step-by-step procedure" to define codes with the material at hand, as well as organising and systematising the codes continuously (ibid.: 185). Mixing these approaches entails using "a coding frame with deductively formed codes and the subsequent inductive coding of all data" (ibid.).

The coding process consists of seven steps, which are not a linear sequence but encompass iteration and feedback loops (Kuckartz 2016: 46). Figure 1 shows the seven steps of the coding process.

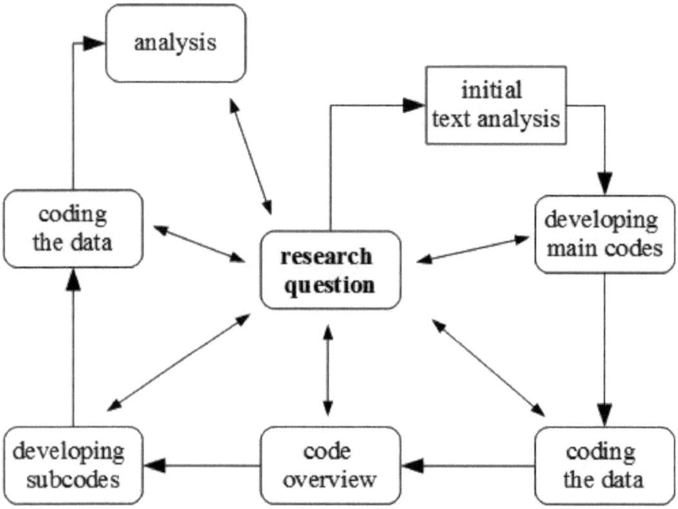

Figure 1: The seven steps of the coding process (Kuckartz/Rädiker 2022)

Research question

At the centre is the research question, which is the basis of the entire process. The research question may be changed, refined and/or adjusted during the research (Kuckartz 2016: 46). The research question, as will be explained below, determines the coding process and therefore the code system. All coding steps are oriented towards the research question.

Initial text analysis

During the first phase – the initial text analysis – the entire text material (e.g. the STs) is read and interesting/striking sections are highlighted. The researcher uses this phase to get a feeling for the material and to develop the first codes (Kuckartz 2016: 101). The software MaxQDA allows researchers to attach "memos" to text segments – i.e. little notes which can be used to attach ideas and thoughts to specific text segments.

Developing the main codes

After reading the material, the main codes are developed using a deductive, inductive, or mixed approach (see above). The main codes have to be clearly defined and differentiated from one another (Kuckartz 2016: 103). For an accessibility-oriented text analysis in intralingual translation, deductively formed main codes could be features of expert language, such as nominalisations, passive voice, and expert terminology – all of which impede perceptibility, comprehensibility, recall, acceptability, and action-enabling potential. Using a mixed method approach can be favourable: text features that are not necessarily characteristic for expert language, and that are thus not deductive codes, can still contribute to communication barriers. These features can be coded inductively and thus still be considered in the text analysis. The *extra-* and *intratextual factors* according to Nord's New Rhetoric Formula can also serve as deductive codes (see Chapter 3.2 and Ahrens in prep.).

Coding the data with the main codes

The main codes are then used to code the entire material (Kuckartz 2016: 102). This means reading every text line by line and assigning codes to relevant segments. The segments need to be coded in a way that they can be understood out of their context as well (ibid. 104), e.g. coding an entire sentence showing passive voice rather than the verb only, as the researcher will work with code overviews rather than the entire text(s) later on (see Chapter 4). Segments of the same category can later be viewed at a glance, without missing the co-text.

Preparing a code overview and developing subcodes

After the material is coded, a code overview needs to be provided. Code overviews are lists of each code and their respective coded segments. These lists are used to develop subcodes inductively for each main code (Kuckartz 2016: 106). The text analysis for intralingual translation may require a reverse process: First the subcodes are developed (e.g. the linguistic features such as passive voice and nominalisations) that are then integrated into broader concepts and main codes (see Chapters 3 and 4). This has a simple reason: Text analysis focuses on specific textual or linguistic features. For an accessibility-oriented text analysis, and to answer the research question, these features need sorting into broader categories, for example the passive and its alternatives (see Chapter 3.1) could be subsumed as agent-hiding features (Ahrens in prep.) or under Nord's *intratextual factor syntax*. This makes a reverse approach necessary, leaving the suggestions from qualitative content analysis behind.

Coding the data

At this point an extensive coding set has been developed which is now used to code the entire material (Kuckartz 2016: 110). Kuckartz (2019: 186) emphasises that "[t]he creation of categories and subcategories and the coding of the data can take place in several cycles." (see Figure 1). Afterwards "a systematization and structuring of all the relevant data in view of the research question at hand will have been achieved" (Kuckartz 2019: 186).

Analysing the coded data

Now, different analyses can be performed. The researcher can examine certain categories in depth as well as analyse individual cases. The researcher may use various methods of data analysis (Kuckartz 2016: 117). This illustrates that qualitative data analysis is only one tool for text analysis which needs to be flanked by other methods (see Chapter 3). Qualitative data analysis offers the possibility of using both inductive and deductive codes to analyse the material. This allows an extensive analysis of the texts. For an accessibility-oriented text analysis, this method offers a structured process, which is especially helpful when analysing *lexis*, *syntax*, pragmatics (e.g. *sender's intention* and *addressees*), and *content* of the source text.

The analysis can be further enriched by the use of other tools, such as TextLab and AntConc. TextLab (H&H Communication Lab 2020) is a software to check the comprehensibility of texts. It can be used to generate data on each text, e.g. number of sentences, average word length and average sentence length, passive voice, abstract nouns, sentence structure, etc., using the "Hohenheimer Verständlichkeitsindex". TextLab is a tool for text producers that indicates overt complexity (Rink in prep.) and allows researchers to make changes to improve comprehensibility (see Zehrer 2019). The free corpus analysis tool AntConc (Laurence Anthony) generates word lists, including the number of types and tokens within the analysed text. These lists can be further developed into word frequency lists, after correcting for homonyms and declinations. Both add specific foci to the analysis that can be combined with the analysis conducted in MaxQDA.

3 Text Analysis in research – reports from two projects

In this paper, we will report on two research projects and how they use the methods and tools described in Chapter 2 to gain insight into the accessibility of health texts. A proposal for an accessibility-oriented text analysis schema for intralingual translation is derived from both approaches. The projects analyse two text types: Kröger (in prep.) analyses information texts on the web about ailments and illnesses. She analyses overall accessibility of the texts taking various features into account that are connected to all steps of the accessibility process. Ahrens (in prep.) analyses a patient information form, partly information text, partly interaction text (see Rink 2020: 125), distributed in print. She analyses the texts with regards to comprehensibility and action-orientation. Both projects analyse texts that have been translated – broadly speaking – with the scopos to remove communication barriers (Deilen/Hansen-Schirra/Maaß 2019: 48).

3.1 Text analysis for identification of text features and barriers

Kröger (in prep.) analyses standard German health information and their Plain Language translations to determine

- features of the text type,
- the communication barriers that these features contribute to,
- and how the Plain Language target texts address them.

The corpus consists of six standard language texts and their Plain Language translations. The texts inform about specific diseases, the symptoms, possible treatments and disease prevention. The analysis was performed using MaxQDA as described in Chapter 2. In this contribution, only the analysis of the standard language texts will be described.

In the analysis, features of expert language (Roelcke 2010) were used as deductive codes. These codes were, for example, nominalisations, passive voice, complex sentence structure (containing sentences with more than one piece of information) and expert terminology. The deductive codes were the starting point of the analysis. While coding the texts using MaxQDA, other important features were discovered and added to the code tree as inductive codes. Inductive codes included sentences in which users were addressed directly and references to affected persons (e.g. patients) (for details on the coding process see Chapter 3.3 and Kröger in prep.). The combination of inductive and deductive codes created a comprehensive picture of the ST features. At the same time, a text analysis using TextLab was conducted to evaluate overt complexity (Rink in prep.). The software was used to gain insight on, among others, average sentence length, use of abstract nouns and average word length. The findings complemented the qualitative analysis with MaxQDA. Using both tools, the researcher could report on overt and covert complexity of the texts (see Rink in prep.).

3.2 *Intratextual factors* of the New Rhetoric Formula as deductive codes

Ahrens (in prep.) examines how Plain Language health texts need to be written in order to be optimally comprehensible and action-oriented for the target group of women with German as a second language (GSL). Her text material consists of a standard language patient information text (cervical biopsy) and its Plain Language translation. The latter will be developed during the research process, consisting of two main versions: one after literature research, the other after an interview study. In this contribution, only the analysis of the standard text (i.e. the ST) will be discussed.

She first analysed the *intratextual factors* according to Nord's New Rhetoric Formula. On this basis, she later analysed the *extratextual factors*, which will not be described in this contribution. Depending on the *intratextual factor*, different methods were used:

For *topic*, *contents* and *structure*, Ahrens used literature that described the legal requirements for patient information materials in Germany (Heberer, Hüttl 2010: 169). She checked whether the required information was contained in the text, and if it followed the prescribed *text structure*.

Non-verbal elements were analysed inductively, without the use of any computer-based tools.

Lexis was first analysed in AntConc which provided a list of all the words contained in the text. Duplicates, e.g. declinations of the same type, were eliminated and homonyms were separated to be counted as different words. From the finished list, a list of potential expert terminology was created with the help of an expert from the health domain. Long words with over 16 letters were identified using the programme TextLab.

Syntax was first analysed in TextLab. Here, sentence length and overall complexity were evaluated. *Syntax* was then more closely examined in MaxQDA. The steps according to qualitative content analysis were applied only to this *intratextual factor*. The features of expert language (derived from literature research, see Chapter 3.1) were used as deductive codes, for example the use of passive constructions. As explained in Chapter 2.3, subcodes were soon found to be the starting point of text analysis with MaxQDA. Thus, features such as modal infinitives with *sein* or light verb constructions (*Funktionsverbgefüge*) were soon coded and evaluated to be equally as inaccessible as passive constructions. All three were thus subsumed under the main code "features that erase the agent". This shows that the deductive codes can change during the iterative coding process, in this case from "use of passive constructions" to "features that erase the agent".

Knowledge presuppositions were analysed after all data from the other seven *intratextual factors* had been evaluated. It was necessary to first analyse *topic*, *contents*, *text structure* as well as the nature of the *non-verbal elements* and of *lexis*, *syntax* and *tone* to determine what prior knowledge the *addressees* need to read the text. Using the same information, the *extratextual factor addressees* was determined. The analysis of *knowledge presuppositions* will be enriched by the outcomes of the empirical user study.

3.3 Accessibility-oriented text analysis: *passive voice*

In this chapter, the process of ST analysis according to the proposed text analysis schema will be explained with the example of the passive voice and passive alternatives (see Pedrini in this volume).

Initial text analysis

Before reading the ST, the researchers were already aware of the features of medical expert language such as usage of complex syntax structures, passive voice, and expert terminology (cf. Roelcke 2010). The medical expert language features were aligned with Nord's New Rhetoric Formula: Nord's *intratextual factor lexis* thus contained features like expert terminology, foreign words and compound nouns, the factor *syntax* contained features like complex syntax structure, passive voice and nominalisations. In the following, we will show the analysis process using the feature *passive voice.*

While reading the ST for the first time, obvious occurrences of the passive voice were marked, showing that this deductive code is applicable to the STs.

Developing the subcodes

The passive-code became one of the first codes in both research projects, alongside other syntax factors like nominalisations or modifiers. As explained in 2.3, for text analysis it was useful to not start with main codes, but with subcodes. For both researchers, the code tree looked like this at this point:

syntax
    nominalisations
    modifiers
    passive voice
    …

Coding the data with the subcodes

Having categorised the passive voice as a subcode of syntax, the text was analysed sentence by sentence to identify instances of passive voice.

Code overview

A table of coded segments was prepared to list all occurrences of passive in the text(s). This is used for the next step.

Developing subcodes – differentiating subcodes

Analysis of the coded segments revealed instances of passive alternatives and doubtful cases of passive. The codes needed to be defined more precisely to make them distinguishable, leading to the creation of the subcode passive alternatives, e.g. *lassen* + infinitive or reflexive constructions. The code was established inductively according to its occurrence in the respective ST.

Like Pedrini (this volume), the researchers found the following passive alternatives in both medical text types:

- ***lassen* + infinitive**
  In Schulungen oder von Ihrem Arzt können sich Asthmatiker solche Haltungen und Techniken zeigen lassen. (Apotheken Umschau 2019)
  Asthma patients can be shown such postures and techniques in training courses or by their doctor. (Translation J. K.)

- **reflexive constructions**
  Danach entscheidet sich, *ob und welche weiteren Behandlungsmaßnahmen notwendig werden.* (Merkle/Schlund 2018: 3)
  Afterwards, it will be decided if and which further treatment measures become necessary. (Translation S. A.)

- ***zu-Infinitiv*: modal infinitives with *sein***
  Auf diese Weise sind Beschwerden gezielt zu lindern. (Apotheken Umschau 2018)
  This way symptoms can be alleviated in a targeted manner. (Translation J. K.)

- ***Funktionsverbgefüge* (light verb constructions)**
  Sofern dies bei Ihnen in Betracht kommt, *werden Sie darüber aufgeklärt.* (Merkle/Schlund 2018: 1)
  If this comes into question for you, you will be informed about it. (Translation S. A.)

Repeating code overview

During and after developing and differentiating the subcodes, it became evident that the code system needed to be rearranged to fit the research question. Thus, an iterative step was needed. The codes relating to the passive voice and passive alternatives, initially categorised as subcodes of syntax, were allocated to main codes that answer the research question more precisely. Kröger identified them as features that indicate distance to the reader (Koch/Oesterreicher 1985) while Ahrens identified them as features that erase the agent in a sentence.

Kröger's code tree had the following form:

features that indicate proximity or distance
- passive
- passive alternatives
- direct ways of addressing the reader

It is evident that codes can be arranged differently. This shows not only the difference in research question, but also the individuality of each text, considering text type, *text function*, and communication situation, including *sender's intention*, *motive for communication* and *addressees*.

Coding the data

In this phase, the researcher searches the ST for each code. This process can be simplified by using the "search" function in MaxQDA (VERBI Software GmbH 2021). In the case of the passive and passive alternatives, it is possible to search for forms of *werden* to find the *Vorgangspassiv*. By searching for *sich*, the researcher can find the reflexive passive alternatives. Using the search function, fewer occurrences will be overlooked. This can complement the line-by-line approach in which each code is traced manually.

Analysing the coded data

In this step, all categories are reviewed to reveal the characteristics of the ST as well as barriers that emerge due to the textual qualities.

Due to the iterative nature of Kuckartz' qualitative content analysis, the described steps can be repeated as necessary (cf. Kuckartz 2016: 46, 186; see Chapter 2.3). This is especially relevant for the rearrangement of subcodes into main codes: The more of Nord's formula is analysed, the more the focus of the ST analysis can change. This becomes apparent when the researcher analyses the passive and passive alternatives in relation to other factors of Nord's New Rhetoric Formula. The passive and its alternatives also play a role in the factors *knowledge presuppositions* and *tone*. The passive voice is notoriously difficult to comprehend (for example Dąbrowska/Street 2006) in part due to its lack of or concealing of the agent. The researcher can thus draw conclusions for *knowledge presuppositions* that the *author* or *sender* suspects the *addressees* to have. A comprehensive use of passive and passive alternatives thus shows that the *author/sender* expects the *addressees* to be strong readers with a thorough ability to infer the lacking or hidden agents from the extra- or intratextual context of the text. It is thus presupposed that readers know how to read well, i.e. are fully literate. This shows the extent of the cognitive, language and expert language barriers within a text. The passive and its alternatives influence the *tone* of a text, too (Ahrens 2020). Hiding the agent is one of the linguistic devices that can be employed to save the reader's negative face (Brown/Levinson 1987: 317), i.e. the reader's "basic want to maintain claims of territory and self-determination" (Brown/Levinson 1987: 317). By hiding the agent, direct requests or demands are veiled and the required or forbidden act is distanced from the reader (Brown/Levinson 1987: 317). The text thus does not overtly impede on the reader's want to self-determination and "[permits] him to feel that his response is not coerced" (Brown/Levinson 1987: 317). This sort of "redressive action" is called "negative politeness" (Brown/Levinson 1987: 317).

In medical communication, removing the agent may serve as a device to remove the reader from potentially emotional subjects. In the following example, life-threatening complications of a disease are mentioned which can lead to strong reactions as the readers may have been diagnosed with the disease. To remove the reader from involvement, passive voice was used:

> *Da in seltenen Fällen ein lebensbedrohlicher Verlauf aufgrund dieser Komplikationen auftreten kann, sollte bei diesen Anzeichen unbedingt ein Arzt* aufgesucht werden. (Kremser 2018)
> Since a life-threatening course can occur in rare cases due to these complications, in case of these symptoms a doctor should be consulted. (Translation J. K.)

Especially topics like complications and risks can provoke fear and rejection of the content, i.e. the emotional barrier, even more so if the reader is at risk of experiencing the text *topic*. Using the passive voice hides the agent and reduces the readers' involvement. The analysis of *tone* allows for conclusions on the *sender's intention*: Is the passive used to save the reader's face or to protect them from potentially emotional subjects? This analysis then shows how the emotion and motivation barriers are addressed in a given ST.

4 Synthesis: A proposal for text analysis in research

Analysing a text with regard to accessible communication means identifying the communication barriers. Having introduced the three models and methods in Chapter 2, this chapter will abstract from the example given in Chapter 3 to outline how to combine the models to achieve an accessibility-oriented analysis schema for intralingual translation with the aim of identifying barriers.

Kuckartz' qualitative content analysis serves as a frame for Nord's New Rhetoric Formula. The New Rhetoric Formula offers factors for the text analysis itself – the qualitative content analysis structures the analysis (see Chapter 2.3). For each factor according to the New Rhetoric Formula, the researcher follows the iterative cycle of Kuckartz' qualitative content analysis. Following this schema, codes are developed according to the factors. It is possible that the factors become codes themselves, or that they are grouped or divided into more suitable main or sub-codes (see Chapters 2.3 and 3.3).

Nord's *extratextual factors* are mostly exempt from this iterative analysis process: They are usually easily analysed from extratextual information. However, *extratextual factors* such as *addressees*, *sender's intention*, or *text function* may not be provided externally, but need to be assessed from the *intratextual factors* (for an example see Chapter 3.3).

Each of Nord's *intratextual factors* undergoes the iterative process of the qualitative content analysis. The factors usually contain sub-factors, such as the passive and passive alternatives as sub-factors of *syntax*. These sub-factors can be deductive or inductive codes that are developed further during each iterative step. They are themselves analysed iteratively which makes the text analysis time-consuming. Using programmes like MaxQDA (VERBI GmbH 2021) can support and help to structure the analysis (see Chapter 3).

A combination of the New Rhetoric Formula and the qualitative content analysis in MaxQDA allows for text analysis in context, i.e. *lexis* can be analysed with regards to the surrounding co-text. Without coding in programmes such as MaxQDA, researchers often rely on frequency lists (Vaughan/O'Keeffe 2015: 5ff.) in which words are counted based on their appearance, not on their semantics (i.e. word class and word function) (see Chapter 3.2). Iterative coding in MaxQDA allows for ongoing semantic analysis where necessary to avoid mistakes in lexical analysis, especially in word (class) frequency analysis. The search function in MaxQDA ensures that no token occurrences are missed.

The last step is the analysis of the coded data (see Chapter 3.3). The coding is performed to determine features of a text, here the factors in Nord's New Rhetoric Formula, which can then be linked to the accessible communication model and to potential communication barriers (see Chapter 2.1). Depending on the research question, the coding can focus on certain factors and the analysis can yield different results.

Nord's *intratextual factors* all potentially impede comprehensibility and linkability (for an initial overview see Chapters 2.2 and 3.3). Depending on the research question, text *topic* and *content* can be identified as part of an expert knowledge barrier, but can also be attributed to a cultural barrier (Ahrens/Fioravanti in prep.), thus affecting comprehensibility and linkability. In TT planning, it is additionally relevant to select information to achieve an acceptable text length (see Chapter 2.2). *Text structure* is guided by text type conventions and thus tied to the expert language barrier and the cultural barrier (Schubert 2016: 18; Rink 2020: 139), affecting comprehensibility and action-orientation. *Non-verbal elements*, in written texts often images, can be attributed to perceptibility, comprehensibility and acceptability. In Ahrens (in prep.) images are interpreted to potentially reduce the expert language barrier by showing the placement of organs within the abdomen, therefore enhancing the ST's comprehensibility. *Lexis* and *syntax*, especially in projects for expert-non-expert communication, can be attributed to the expert language barrier, but also to the language barrier, affecting perceptibility and comprehensibility. *Tone* has been attributed to the emotional and motivational barrier in Chapter 2.2, and thus affects acceptability. The passive voice may have a positive impact on acceptability by saving the reader's face or removing the reader from the text *topic* (see Chapter 3.3). *Knowledge presuppositions* affect the stages of comprehensibility, linkability and acceptability as they not only play a potential role in the expert knowledge barrier, but also in the cultural barrier (Ahrens/Fioravanti in prep.) and the motivational barrier. Hiding the agent with a passive construction, for example, implies that the text presupposes that the reader knows the agent already or can infer the agent easily (see Chapter 3.3). Counting literacy and numeracy into the factor *knowledge presuppositions*, the cognitive and language barrier might also be identified.

Extratextual factors such as *sender*, *author*, and *sender's intention* relate to acceptability (see Chapter 2.2). Health information distributed by state-funded health institutions can be more trustworthy than health information distributed by ad-driven companies (Sun et al. 2019: 11; Deutsches Netzwerk evidenzbasierte Medizin e.V. 2017; for a study on health information searches on the web see for example Zschorlich et al. 2015), hence more acceptable (Lang 2021: 101; for trust in health information see Link 2019: 108).

Sender and *author*, however, could also relate to retrievability. Especially during the Covid-19 pandemic, readers might have memorised senders such as the *Robert Koch Institut* (a state-funded health institution in Germany) or authors such as popular virologists. Knowledge of these names helps them look for reliable health information (for issues with the retrievability of reliable health information see for example Schaeffer et al. 2016: 59f., 2021: 26; Zschorlich et al. 2015). More poignant examples are found in literature when readers search for books by a specific author: The books become more retrievable when the author's name is attached to them.

Having analysed Nord's *intratextual factors*, conclusions about unanalysed *extratextual factors* can be drawn (see above). For example: *Knowledge presuppositions* that were made in the text hint at the *addressees* and the *sender's intention*.

These examples show that the New Rhetoric Formula can conveniently be used to analyse the accessibility of a text, the iterative process of the qualitative content analysis ensuring a thorough, high-quality analysis.

As shown in Chapter 3.2, the process according to the qualitative content analysis can also serve to complete a text analysis that is framed by the New Rhetoric Formula. Here, it may only be used to analyse one of the *intralingual factors*, in this case *syntax*. This procedure may be advisable for research projects in which the text analysis has a minor role.

5 Conclusion

In this paper we have shown how to conduct an accessibility-oriented, research-focussed text analysis. We have shown how the New Rhetoric Formula, designed for interlingual translation, can serve in intralingual translation research, too. Thirdly, we have demonstrated how to conduct a thorough text analysis using the tool MaxQDA, following the iterative steps of qualitative content analysis. The combination of the factors in Nord's New Rhetoric Formula and the iterative framework provided by Kuckartz' qualitative content analysis allows for an intensive analysis of a source text with a large spectrum of codes oriented at the given research question. The research questions guide the analysis of the data to interpret their influence on the communication barriers, and thus on the steps retrievability, perceptibility, comprehensibility, linkability, acceptability, and action-orientation. Using software like MaxQDA helps the coding process and prevents text segments from being missed.

This contribution attempts to further the field of intralingual translation studies as part of translation studies by adapting translation theories to intralingual translation. We show how interdisciplinary research can support research projects and how it can help to improve how we research.

Literature

Ahrens, Sarah (2020): "Easy Language and Administrative Texts: Second Language Learners as a Target Group." In: Silvia Hansen-Schirra/Christiane Maaß (Hg.): *Easy language research: text and user perspectives* (Easy – Plain – Accessible), pp. 67–97.

Ahrens, Sarah/Fioravanti, Chiara (in prep.): "Cultural implications in Easy Language texts for migrants: theoretical considerations and insights from practice in Germany and in Italy". In: Deilen, Silvana/Hansen-Schirra, Silvia/Hernández Garrido, Sergio/Maaß, Christiane/Tardel, Anke (eds.): *Easy Language and Accessible Communication.*

Anthony, Laurence (2022): AntConc (Version 4.0.11) [Computer Software]. Tokyo, Japan: Waseda University. Available from https://www.laurenceanthony.net/software.

Apotheken Umschau (2018): *Parkinson-Krankheit: Symptome, Ursachen , Therapie.* https://www.apotheken-umschau.de/krankheiten-symptome/neurologische-erkrankungen/parkinson-krankheit-symptome-ursachen-therapie-733737.html aktualisiert am 17.12.2018

Apotheken Umschau (2019): *Asthma*. https://www.apotheken-umschau.de/krankheiten-symptome/atemwegserkrankungen/asthma-736647.html aktualisiert am 07.06.2019

Bredel, Ursula/Maaß, Christiane (2016): *Leichte Sprache: Theoretische Grundlagen, Orientierung für die Praxis*. Berlin: Dudenverlag.

Brown, Penelope/Levinson, Stephen C. (1987): *Politeness: Some universals in language usage*. Cambridge: Cambridge University Press.

Dąbrowska, Ewa/Street, James (2006): "Individual differences in language attainment: Comprehension of passive sentences by native and non-native English speakers." In: *Language Sciences* 28 (6), pp. 604–615.

Deilen, Silvana/Hansen-Schirra, Silvia/Maaß, Christiane (2019): "Anwendbarkeit der ISO 17100 auf intralinguales Übersetzen in Leichte und Einfache Sprache." In: *mAGAzin Revista intercultural e interdisciplinar* 27, pp. 43–53.

Deutsches Netzwerk Evidenzbasierte Medizin e. V. (2016): *Gute Praxis Gesundheitsinformation: Ein Positionspapier des Deutschen Netzwerks Evidenzbasierte Medizin e.V*. Version 2.0. Berlin.

Früh, Werner (2004): *Inhaltsanalyse. Theorie und Praxis*. 5. Aufl. Konstanz: UVK.

Grice, Herbert Paul (1975): "Logic and conversation." In: Cole, Peter/Morgan, Jerry L. (ed.): *Syntax and Semantics*. Vol. 3. Speech Acts. New York: Academic Press, pp. 41–58.

H&H Communication Lab (2020): TextLab. URL: https://www.comlab-ulm.de/textlab-software/ (last accessed 15th June 2022).

Hansen-Schirra, Silvia/Maaß, Christiane (2019): Translation proper: Kommunikationsbarrieren abbauen. Uni Hildesheim.

Inhoff, Albrecht W./Radach, Ralph/Heller, Dieter (2000): "Complex Compounds in German: Interword Spaces Facilitate Segmentation but Hinder Assignment of Meaning." In: *Journal of Memory and Language* 42 (1), pp. 23–50.

Koch, Peter/Oesterreicher, Wulf (1986): "Sprache der Nähe – Sprache der Distanz: Mündlichkeit und Schriftlichkeit im Spannungsfeld von Sprachtheorie und Sprachgeschichte." In: Deutschmann, Olaf/Flasche, Hans/König, Bernhard/Kruse, Margot/Pabst, Walter/Stempel, Wolf-Dieter (eds.): *Romanistisches Jahrbuch*. Berlin, New York: De Gruyter, pp. 15–43.

Kremser, Katharina (2018): *Neurodermitis. Symptome und Behandlung.* https://www.apotheken-umschau.de/krankheiten-symptome/hautkrankheiten/neurodermitis-symptome-und-behandlung-734571.html aktualisiert am 17.05.2018

Kuckartz, Udo (2016): *Qualitative Inhaltsanalyse. Methoden, Praxis, Computerunterstützung.* 4. Auflage. Weinheim, Basel: Beltz Juventa.

Kuckartz, Udo (2019): "Qualitative Text Analysis: A Systematic Approach." In: Kaiser, G./Presmeg, N. (eds.): *Compendium for early Career Researchers in Mathematics Education*. ICME-13 Monographs.

Lang, Katrin (2021): *Auffindbarkeit, Wahrnehmbarkeit, Akzeptabilität. Webseiten von Behörden in Leichter Sprache vor dem Hintergrund der rechtlichen Lage.* Berlin: Frank & Timme.

Lázaro Gutiérrez, Raquel (2017): "Healthcare Videos Addressed to the Migrant Population. From Intercultural Mediation to Transcreation." In: *Revista de Lenguas para Fines Específicos* 23 (1), pp. 140–162.

Maaß, Christiane (2020): *Easy Language – Plain Language – Easy Language Plus. Balancing Comprehensibility and Acceptability*. Berlin: Frank & Timme. Easy – Plain – Accessible Vol. 3.

Maaß, Christiane/Rink, Isabel (2019): "Über das Handbuch Barrierefreie Kommunikation." In: Maaß, Christiane/Rink, Isabel (Hrsg.): *Handbuch Barrierefreie Kommunikation.* Berlin: Frank & Timme. (Kommunikation – Partizipation – Inklusion), pp. 17–25.

Maaß, Christiane/Rink, Isabel (2020): "Scenarios for Easy Language Translation: How to Produce Accessible Content for Users with Diverse Needs." In: Silvia Hansen-Schirra/Christiane Maaß (eds.): *Easy Language Research: Text and User Perspectives.* Berlin: Frank & Timme. Easy – Plain – Accessible Vol. 2. pp. 41–56.

Merkle, Elisabeth/Schlund Gerhard H. (2018): *Eingriffe am Gebärmutterhals. Konisation/Kürettage/Gewebeentnahme*. Erlangen: Thieme Compliance.

Nord, Christiane (1992): “Text Analysis in Translator Training.” In: Dollerup, Cay/Loddegaard, Anne (eds.): *Teaching Translation and Interpreting. Training, Talent and Experience. Papers from the First Language International Conference.* Elsinore (Denmark), 31st May-2nd June 1991. Amsterdam, Philadelphia: John Benjamins Publishing Company (Copenhagen Studies in Translation), pp. 39–48.

Nord, Christiane (2009): *Textanalyse und Übersetzen. Theoretische Grundlagen, Methode und didaktische Anwendung einer übersetzungsrelevanten Textanalyse.* 4th revised edition. Tübingen: Groos.

Rink, Isabel (2019): “Kommunikationsbarrieren.” In: Maaß, Christiane/Rink, Isabel (eds.): *Handbuch Barrierefreie Kommunikation*. Berlin: Frank & Timme (Kommunikation – Partizipation – Inklusion, Band 3), pp. 29–65.

Rink, Isabel (2020): *Rechtskommunikation und Barrierefreiheit. Zur Übersetzung juristischer Informations- und Interaktionstexte in Leichte Sprache*. Berlin: Frank & Timme. Easy – Plain – Accessible Vol. 01

Rink, Isabel (in prep.): “Competences for Easy Language translation.” In: Deilen, Silvana/Hansen-Schirra, Silvia/Hernández Garrido, Sergio/Maaß, Christiane/Tardel, Anke (eds.): *Easy Language and Accessible Communication.*

Schaeffer, Doris/Vogt, Dominique/Berens, Eva-Maria/Hurrelmann, Klaus (2016): *Gesundheitskompetenz der Bevölkerung in Deutschland: Ergebnisbericht.* Bielefeld. URL: <https://doi.org/10.2390/0070-pub-29081112> (last accessed 25.11.2021).

Schaeffer, Doris/Berens, Eva.-Maria/Gille, Svea/Griese, Lennert/Klinger, Julia/de Sombre, Steffen/Vogt, Dominique/Hurrelmann, Klaus (2021): *Gesundheitskompetenz der Bevölkerung in Deutschland – vor und während der Corona Pandemie: Ergebnisse des HLS-GER 2*. Bielefeld: Interdisziplinäres Zentrum für Gesundheitskompetenz-forschung (IZGK), Universität Bielefeld. DOI: <https://doi.org/10.4119/unibi/2950305> (last accessed 25.11.2021).

Schubert, Klaus (2016): “Barriereabbau durch optimierte Kommunikationsmittel: Versuch einer Systematisierung”. In: Mälzer, Nathalie (ed.): *Barrierefreie Kommunikation – Perspektiven aus Theorie und Praxis*. Berlin: Frank & Timme, pp. 15–33.

Sun, Yalin/Zhang, Yan/Gwizdka, Jacek/Trace, Ciaran B. (2019): "Consumer Evaluation of the Quality of Online Health Information: Systematic Literature Review of Relevant Criteria and Indicators." In: *Journal of medical Internet research* 21 (5), e12522.

Vaughan, Elaine/O'Keeffe, Anne (2015): "Corpus Analysis." In: Tracy, Karen (ed.): *The international encyclopedia of language and social interaction.* Chichester: Wiley-Blackwell, 1–17. URL: <https://onlinelibrary.wiley.com/doi/full/10.1002/9781118611463.wbielsi168> (last accessed: 24.11.2021).

VERBI Software GmbH (2020): MAXQDA Analytics Pro 2020 Students. URL: <https://www.maxqda.de/produkte/maxqda-analytics-pro> (last accessed: 25.11.2021).

Zehrer, Christiane (2019): "Schreib- und Übersetzungswerkzeuge für die Barrierefreie Kommunikation." In: Maaß, Christiane/Rink, Isabel (eds.): *Handbuch Barrierefreie Kommunikation*. Berlin: Frank & Timme.

Zschorlich, Beate/Gechter, Dorothea/Janssen, Inger M./Swinehart, Thomas/Wiegard, Beate/Koch, Klaus (2015): "Gesundheitsinformationen im Internet: Wer sucht was, wann und wie?" In: *Zeitschrift für Evidenz, Fortbildung und Qualitat im Gesundheitswesen* 109 (2), pp. 144–152.

Kristin Leyerer / Anja Tüchler /
Rita Schmutzler / Susanne Weg-Remers

Providing Evidence-Based Health Information in Easy and Plain Language

Procedures and Experiences of the Cancer Information Service

1 Introduction

The Cancer Information Service (CIS) of the German Cancer Research Center is a publicly funded institution dedicated to providing evidence-based information on cancer to the public. People can ask their individual questions about the disease by telephone and email. This service is flanked by a website (www.krebsinformationsdienst.de) providing profound online information and print materials such as brochures and leaflets on selected topics.

The offer of CIS is aimed at patients, their relatives, or anyone interested in knowing more about cancer. Topics on the website range from general information on prevention, screening, diagnostic procedures, and cancer therapies to specific information for the most frequent cancer entities, and on life with cancer. Individual inquiries are answered by specially trained physicians by telephone or email, based on a comprehensive evidence-based knowledge database that is regularly updated.

In addition, CIS provides information for healthcare professionals through its different channels. This includes physicians, pharmacists, psychologists, nurses and others involved in the treatment and care of cancer patients.

To reach groups with low health literacy in particular, the portfolio of CIS is continually expanded by easy-to-understand information. This includes information in Easy Language and Plain Language. By enhancing the comprehensibility of materials, CIS aims to improve the support of target groups with low health literacy. For example, as part of the EU-funded project "iPAAC", CIS is developing brochures on familial breast and ovarian cancer in cooperation with the Center for Familial Breast and Ovarian Cancer (CC-HBOC) at the University Hospital Cologne. Different brochures will be addressed to at-risk patients and relatives with different levels of health literacy, as well as physicians involved in the counselling and treatment of these families.

2 Motivation for Easy Language Information

Recently, the German Health Literacy Survey (HLS) has observed that about two thirds of the German-speaking population have only limited, self-reported health literacy (Schaeffer et al. 2021). That means that a major share of the general public experiences difficulties in accessing, understanding, appraising, and applying health information to their own condition (Sørensen et al. 2012). Health literacy even seems to have deteriorated, as compared to a first survey conducted in 2014 (Schaeffer et al. 2016). The authors of the study discuss, among other factors, an increasingly complex healthcare system, digitalisation, and fake news and conspiracy myths as potential influencing factors. Although overall health literacy increased slightly during the COVID-19 pandemic (Schaeffer et al. 2021), this remains a major issue that needs to be considered in health communication and health care.

One obstacle in understanding health-related information can be limited reading abilities. The "LEO" study[1], conducted in Germany in 2018, found that 12.1 % of the German-speaking population has problems reading longer sentences or texts (Grotlüschen et al. 2019). Low literacy was also found to be associated with deficits in dealing with health-related texts, e.g., medication package inserts (Grotlüschen et al. 2019).

As stated before, the aim of CIS is to provide information for everyone with questions about cancer. However, recent surveys of CIS users[2] have shown that

1 The LEO study examined literacy in the German-speaking population. Reading and writing skills were assessed among 7,192 participants aged 18–64 years. The study was representative of the German population.

2 Shown by internal polls among users of the services, non-representative; results are unpublished.

the CIS website, and also telephone and email services are primarily used by advice-seeking people with higher education. Also, inquirers contacting CIS are mostly actively seeking health information and demonstrate high interest in health topics (Rosset et al. 2019). One reason for that might be the overall complexity and accessibility of the online and print information. A possible measure to address this issue is to improve accessibility of materials and thus provide low-threshold access. One important step in this context is the development of comprehensible brochures in Easy Language and a particular graphic and layout design supporting perceptibility. In the following paragraphs, Easy and Plain Language projects will be presented in more detail.

3 Project Design: Brochures in Easy Language

Easy Language is a very simplified German language that can be helpful for everyone who has trouble understanding Standard German texts (Netzwerk Leichte Sprache 2021, Bredel/Maaß 2016). Thus, the authors have identified Easy Language as one approach to reach new target groups. Easy Language can be used to address people with learning and/or reading disabilities. Visually or hearing impaired people can also benefit from Easy Language. Furthermore, people who are not native speakers and have only a limited speech intelligibility may be recipients of Easy Language texts, as well as people suffering from cognitive impairments and elderly people (Hansen-Schirra/Maaß 2020: 25).

Easy Language has strict rules. Its characteristics include use of very short sentences, extensive explanations of concepts considered little known, additional illustrations of texts, and lack of technical terms, to name a few (Netzwerk Leichte Sprache 2021; Maaß 2015). Transferring health information into such a format requires simplifications and reduction of content (Bredel/Maaß 2016; Maaß/Rink 2017). Thus, the key challenge is to keep evidence-based information easy to understand, and still compliant with common standards for evidence-based health information (Arbeitsgruppe GPGI 2016). Figure 1 shows some of the important aspects to consider.

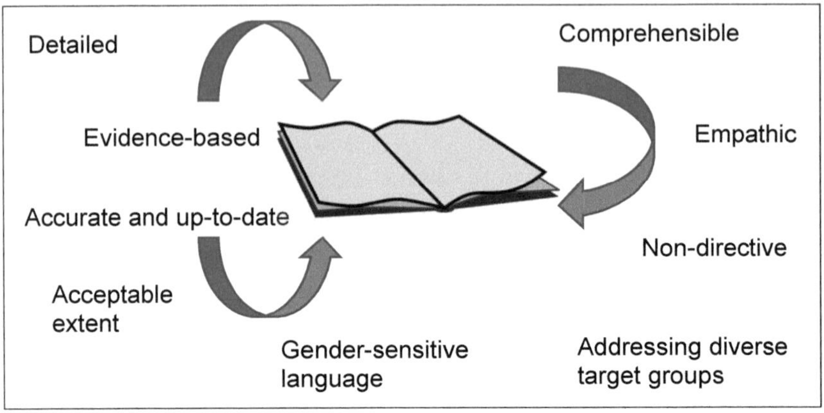

Figure 1: Requirements identified for health information.

It is challenging to balance comprehensibility of Easy Language materials without distortion of the basic facts and information, since Easy Language requires simplifications and truncations. In addition, a certain depth of detail is required while maintaining an acceptable length, which can be difficult due to the extensive explanations needed in Easy Language (Maaß/Rink 2020).

With respect to the frequently vulnerable groups, e.g., cancer patients and their relatives, who are potential users of Easy Language materials, it is important that texts reflect empathy and use a gender-sensitive language. In the cancer healthcare setting, decisive and preference-sensitive medical decisions must frequently be made. Thus, it is mandatory to use a non-directive language which opens spaces for decisions rather than prescribing certain decisions to the reader.

4 Producing Easy Language and Plain Language Health Information

This chapter focuses on health information in Easy Language, describing pilot projects that have set the framework for Easy Language materials at the Cancer Information Service (Chapter 4.1). Afterwards, a closer look will be taken at the production of health information on the complex topic of familial breast and ovarian cancer at different language levels (Chapter 4.2).

4.1 Pilot: Lung Cancer Brochure and Cancer Prevention Brochure

In 2014, CIS started working on brochures in Easy Language in a cooperation between CIS and Prof. Dr. Karin Terfloth of Heidelberg University of Education and her students. As term papers, students wrote manuscripts for brochures on a self-chosen cancer topic in Easy Language, supported by a CIS expert for the respective field. So far, two manuscripts have been illustrated and laid out and subsequently published as brochures of the CIS: "Lungen·krebs – was nun?" (*Lung cancer – what now?*) (Betz et al. 2017) and "Gute Tipps für ein kleineres Krebs·risiko" (*Good advice for a lower cancer risk*) (Barber et al. 2022).

Lung cancer brochure

During the development of the first brochure on lung cancer, focus group tests in the target group were conducted. The target group consisted of 24 participants who were students receiving special needs education and 24 participants who worked at sheltered workshops. All exhibited reading difficulties. The participants read two excerpts in different layouts from the brochure. On that basis, comprehensibility of text and illustrations of the two versions were tested, and participants were interviewed about handling of and orientation within the brochure. Full proceedings of the focus group tests are reported in (Klein et al. 2020).

The focus group tests showed:

- the use of a narrative protagonist was beneficial for understanding
- illustrations and photos were equally well understood
- illustrations were required throughout the brochure, also for table of contents and glossary

These insights were considered in a revision of the manuscript and in the final layout of the brochure. One decision was to use illustrations instead of photos

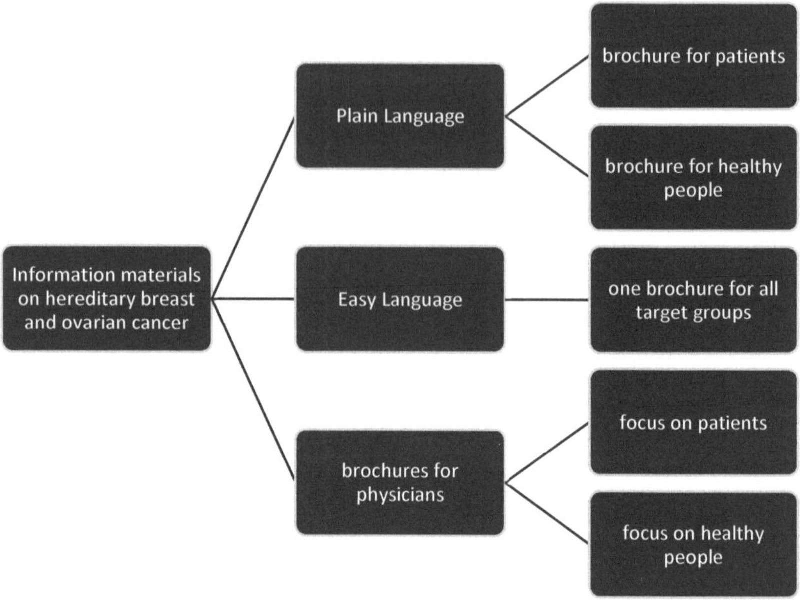

Figure 3: Overview of brochures on familial breast and ovarian cancer developed in the project "iPAAC".

Easy Language brochure

For the Easy Language brochure on familial breast and ovarian cancer, the relevant topics were selected by CIS and CC-HBOC in a first step. Since the focus was supposed to be on genetic predisposition and genetic testing, the principles of heredity needed to be described. Each chapter in the brochure was dedicated to one central aspect in the context of familial breast and ovarian cancer (Table 1). They covered a basic introduction to the topic, as well as possible consequences of a positive genetic test, including options for cancer prevention and early detection. To provide information for patients already suffering from breast or ovarian cancer, two chapters were focused on treatment options and aftercare.

Chapter	Central question / idea	Content
1	Ms. Müller suffers from breast cancer.	Introduction of the narrative
2	What is breast and ovarian cancer?	Basics, carcinogenesis, frequency of breast and ovarian cancer
3	What does heredity mean?	Definition of genes and heredity, introduction of the concept "genetic predisposition"
4	How does genetic testing work?	Procedure and possible outcomes of a genetic test, advantages and disadvantages
5	How can cancer be diagnosed?	Screening and early detection programme for breast cancer, description of screening methods
6	How can cancer be treated?	Description of common cancer therapies
7	What happens after cancer treatment?	Aftercare and rehabilitation, palliative situation
8	What can you do to prevent hereditary cancer?	Introduction of the concept "prevention", preventive mastectomy and removal of ovaries

Table 1: Central questions for chapters in Easy Language brochure on familial breast and ovarian cancer

The main body of the brochure is accompanied by an introductory section explaining how the brochure works and a glossary with explanations of some technical terms and complex concepts.

Regarding the requirements in Figure 1, the following paragraphs present some strategies executed to meet them.

Complexity vs. comprehensibility

To deal with the challenge of making complex information understandable, all texts were edited by internal experts from CIS and CC-HBOC to make sure that all important medical aspects were considered and presented in a correct way. Still, information was only presented to a certain level of detail. For example, the part on possible options for prevention was left quite vague and pointed the reader to a personal consultation with his or her physician. This was partly motivated by the complexity of the topic, but also by conceptional reasons, because prevention options like surgical breast removal requires counselling and support of healthcare professionals, and this cannot be replaced by written information in a brochure.

Narrative

For this brochure, a narrative was used, similar to the lung cancer brochure (see above). Here, the topic is introduced with a sample family, where "Ms. Müller" suffers from breast cancer and her two daughters are confronted with their own potential cancer risk.

As the narrative used in the lung cancer brochure was conducive to comprehensibility (Klein et al. 2020), it was decided to implement a narrative in the new brochure too. Here, its purpose is not only to enhance comprehensibility, but also to offer figures of identification for different target groups. Patients could relate to breast cancer patient Ms. Müller, whereas relatives might identify themselves with the daughters, or her husband, Mr. Müller.

It should be noted that narratives are often viewed critically in health communication due to the risk of generalisation of single, subjective perspectives and thus potential bias in medical decision making (Winterbottom et al. 2008). In the German Guideline Evidence-based Health Information, the use of narratives is not recommended because of potential effects of persuasiveness (Lühnen et al. 2017). Still, the evidence for adverse effects of narratives is rather low, leading to the recommendation of a cautious use of narratives in patient information such as decision aids (Shaffer et al. 2021).

Furthermore, the narrative in this brochure differs from "classical" narratives: It is not a patient story or experience, but a stylistic device to make the topic more tangible for the reader. Nevertheless, strategies were implemented to address the potential issues a narrative can have. First of all, a disclaimer was included at the beginning of the brochure to explain the narrative concept. The disclaimer explicitly states the exemplary status of the narrative (Table 2).

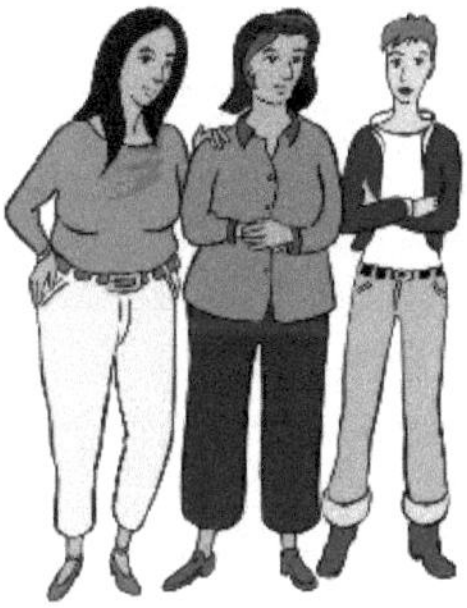	In diesem Heft gibt es die Geschichte von Frau Müller und ihren Töchtern Johanna und Lena. Die Geschichte ist nur ein Beispiel. Das Beispiel hilft uns, viele Dinge besser zu erklären. Das bedeutet für Sie: • Vielleicht ist bei Ihnen die Situation genauso wie bei Familie Müller. • Vielleicht ist Ihre Situation aber ganz anders als bei Familie Müller. • Sie müssen sich **nicht** genauso verhalten wie Frau Müller oder ihre Töchter. • Sie treffen vielleicht andere Entscheidungen.
In this brochure, there is the story of Ms. Müller and her daughters. The story is just an example. • The example helps us to explain many things in a better way. • That means for you: • Maybe your situation is the same as the one of the Müller family. • Maybe your situation is completely different from the one of the Müller family. • You do **not** have to act exactly like Ms. Müller or her daughters. • You can make different decisions.	

Table 2: Example – introduction of the narrative

For topics involving decisions, the brochure switches to addressing the reader personally. This is to emphasise that decisions are individual, as shown in the example below for the decision on genetic testing (Table 3).

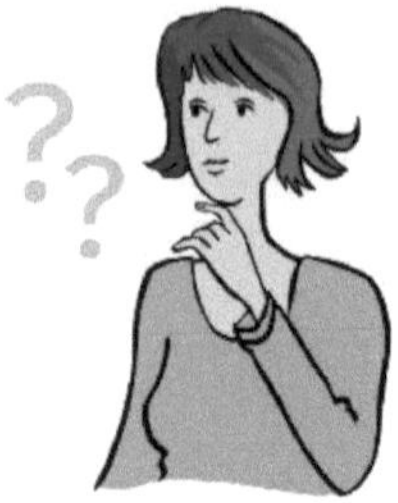 **Denken Sie auch über einen Gen•test nach?** Die Entscheidung ist vielleicht schwierig. Denn der Gen•test hat Vorteile und Nachteile. Es gibt keine richtige oder falsche Entscheidung. Auf der nächsten Seite stehen ein paar Vorteile und Nachteile vom Gen•test. Überlegen Sie gut: Was ist für Sie wichtig?
Are you too thinking about a genetic test? The decision can be difficult. Because the genetic test has advantages and disadvantages. There is no right or wrong decision. On the next page are some advantages and disadvantages of the genetic test. Think carefully: What is important to you?

Table 3: Example – addressing the reader personally

Within the narrative, one daughter decides to take a genetic test, whereas the other daughter decides against it to show that both points of view and resulting decisions are valid and acceptable. Such a decision was needed for the later chapters on screening and prevention to make sense.

Gender-sensitive language

In the German language area, there is a current debate on the use of gender-sensitive language. While the English "patients" applies to men and women, there is a distinction in German between "Patienten" (male patients) and "Patientinnen" (female patients). Apart from naming both individually, there are also special ways of spelling to indicate that all genders are addressed (e.g. "Patient:innen" or "Patient*innen").

This is particularly difficult in Easy Language, as special forms or mentioning of both male and female form make a text more complicated to read

(Rocktäschel 2020). Still, it was important not to use the masculine plural form only, because breast and ovarian cancer affect women, except for a few men suffering from breast cancer. In addition, men should be addressed because they can also inherit a genetic predisposition and pass it on to their children, and be at a higher risk for cancer themselves. As a compromise, a female doctor was included in the narrative, and both forms were used most of the time when general statements were made. In addition, this concept was explained via a disclaimer in the introductory section of the brochure (Table 4).

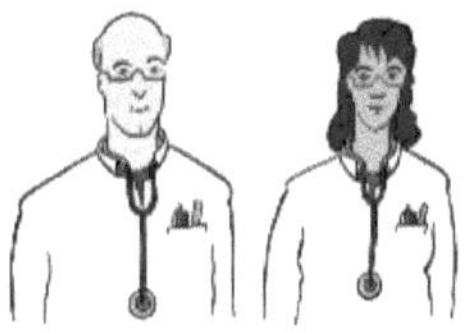	In unserem Beispiel geht Frau Müller zu einer Ärztin. Frau Müller kann natürlich auch zu einem Arzt gehen. Wir meinen alle Menschen mit diesem Beruf. Egal, welches Geschlecht ein Mensch hat.
In our example, Ms. Müller goes to a female doctor. Ms. Müller can of course also go to a male doctor. We mean all people with this profession. No matter what gender a person has.	

Table 4: Disclaimer for gender-sensitive language

Similarly to the other Easy Language brochures, the brochure was illustrated by Reinhild Kassing (including illustrations shown in Figure 2 and Tables 2–4), and comprehensibility of text and layout were checked and approved as paid contract work by test readers at the "Büro für Leichte Sprache" Heidelberg.

Plain Language brochures

For the brochures in Plain Language, it took some time to figure out how to define "Plain Language", as it lacks a set of rules and is more dynamic (Maaß 2020: 150). It is more complex than Easy Language, and requires better reading abilities and a wider knowledge of words and terms (Kellermann 2014).

Initially, Easy Language Plus was supposed to be used, a concept developed by C. Maaß as a language form that balances out the drawbacks of Easy Language and Plain Language (Maaß 2020). In an online user survey, a short text sample in Easy Language Plus was shown to potential readers, followed by administration of a questionnaire asking for their experiences with the text. The text was perceived as easy to understand and well-structured, but some participants missed more detailed information (cf. Figure 4). In the comment section, the text received mixed feedback from the participants of the survey, with some people stating the language was too easy and that the text seemed superficial while others liked the easy-to-understand style.

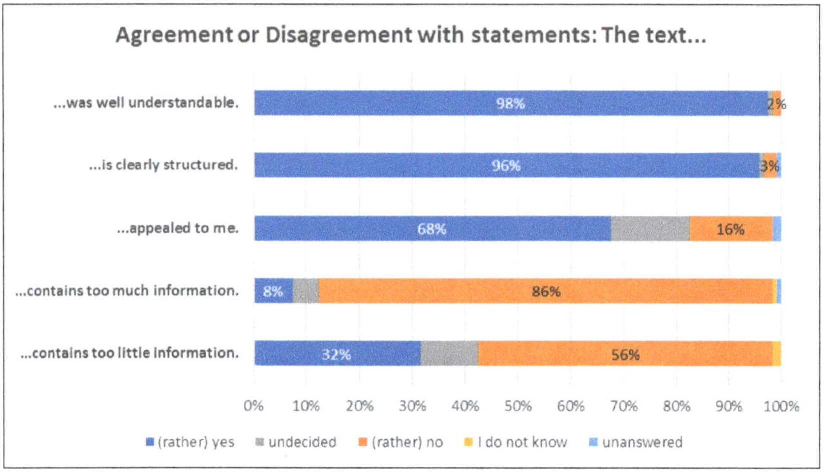

Figure 4: Selected items of a survey on an Easy Language Plus text example (n = 120).

During text production, a switch to a more complex language was made to clearly distinguish these two brochures from the Easy Language text and to present the content in more detail, which turned out to be difficult in Easy Language Plus. Still, the aim was to keep the language relatively simple, e.g., by using only few technical terms and avoiding too lengthy sentences. To enhance understanding, it was decided to use infographics to illustrate the text, as a visual supplement or alternative to the written information. Figure 5 shows an example in which the breast cancer risk for women is presented in a visual form to make frequencies and risks easier to understand.

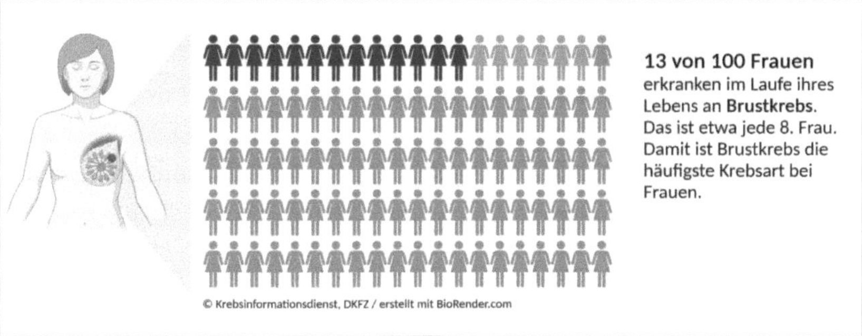

Figure 5: Infographic used for risk communication, showing that 13 out of 100 women develop breast cancer. (Caption: 13 out of 100 women will develop breast cancer in the course of their lives. That is about 1 in 8 women. This makes breast cancer the most common type of cancer in women.)

Prior to finalising and publishing the brochures, structured interviews will be conducted to evaluate whether the text, structure, graphical style and layout are well-received. For the interviews, representatives of the target group will be recruited, i.e., patients seeking advice at the Center for Familial Breast and Ovarian Cancer (CC-HBOC) at the University Hospital Cologne. Also, patient representatives from the patient organisation BRCA Netzwerk e.V. will be asked to review the brochures from the patient's point of view. Their feedback will then be implemented in the finalisation of the brochures prior to publication.

Brochures for physicians

The information materials for patients are accompanied by brochures aimed at health professionals, such as gynaecologists and general practitioners (GPs). Health professionals play an important role in identifying individuals at elevated risk for hereditary cancer, and providing medical information, thus supporting them in medical decision making, e.g., on genetic testing and risk management options. However, evidence-based knowledge on familial breast and ovarian cancer is extensive, complex, and evolves quickly. For health professionals with limited knowledge on genetics, it is a challenge to gain an overview of the current medical evidence, to comprehend the results from molecular genetic analysis, and to translate them into clinical recommendations to support decision making.

As a result, individuals at risk for developing breast and ovarian cancer may not be reliably identified as such by their attending general practitioner, and will subsequently not be sufficiently informed and, if applicable, referred to specialised centres. In addition, patients may receive conflicting medical information by their GPs or gynaecologists, and specialised centres for breast and ovarian cancer (Fadda et al. 2020). This may result in confusion (Nagler et al. 2019; Fadda et al. 2020) and insecurity in medical decisions. Finally, contradictory medical information could even lead to distrust in academic medicine. A cross-sectional survey among German physicians indicated lack of genetic and risk literacy to be a major barrier to routinely discussing genetic issues with patients (Dick et al. 2021). Comprehensible information material on hereditary breast and ovarian cancer for health professionals may assist GPs in identifying and communicating genetic risks (Nippert et al. 2014).

In light of these challenges, the rationale for developing complementary information material was to support health practitioners in identifying and counselling individuals at increased risk for breast and ovarian cancer. The brochures were developed under the lead of CC-HBOC alongside the patient materials produced under the lead of CIS to mirror and complement the information given there.

A health professional's role in enabling preference-sensitive decision making

The health professional's role in the process of decision making is nuanced and unusual in the context of hereditary cancer syndromes. It is characterised by a special prevention situation that is best described by the example of women that are at high risk of developing breast and ovarian cancer, (e.g., due to a pathogenic variant in the *BRCA1* or *BRCA2* gene), but have not (yet) developed the disease. For example, of 100 women with a pathogenic variant in the *BRCA1* gene, around 70 will develop breast cancer during their lifetime, compared to around 12 of 100 women in the general female population (Kuchenbaecker et al. 2017). These women have a clinical indication for prophylactic operations, i.e., bilateral salpingo-oophorectomy (removal of both ovaries and fallopian tubes) and bilateral mastectomy (removal of both breasts). Women deciding on preventive options will face the difficult task of anticipating regret of (not) decision making in light of their lifetime risks. In the example of *BRCA1*, 30 of 100 women will not develop breast cancer during the course of their life. Thus, not opting for a prophylactic measure needs to be considered as a legitimate and important option by health professionals, especially for healthy individuals at risk. These women benefit from health professionals being aware and empathic of their situation, sensitive for counselees' personal preferences and values, as well as their psychosocial situation and life plans – along with evidence-based medical facts as the core and basis for any consultation with individuals at risk.

Structure and contents

The brochures aim to disseminate comprehensive but concise information on the topic of familial cancer to a wider professional audience. This includes an overview on the current state of science on genetic analyses in the context of familial breast and ovarian cancer and their clinical implications. Here, too, the challenge was to find a balance between complexity (in favour of accurate reproduction of scientific and medical facts) and reduction to the essentials (in favour of comprehensibility). In addition, evidence on well-balanced risk communication was incorporated to strengthen a health professional's ability to interpret risks (e.g., the risk of developing breast cancer) and to translate them into clinical recommendations that correspond with the counselee's current situation, age, future plans, personality and values (e.g., future plans on having children) (Gigerenzer et al. 2007). For this, evidence on psychosocial burden and challenges that individuals at risk for breast and ovarian cancer face was considered (Howard et al. 2009). This includes – among many – the loss of close relatives, and the insecurity of if, how, and when to decide on risk management options. An overview of the contents discussed in the brochure for physicians counselling cancer-unaffected individuals at risk is displayed in Table 5.

	Main topics
1	Introduction
2	The German Consortium for Familial Breast and Ovarian Cancer
3	Familial breast and ovarian cancer
4	Offer and procedure of a consultation for genetic testing
5	The process of molecular genetic analyses
6	Interpreting the results of molecular genetic analyses
7	Understanding risks
8	Clinical consequences following genetic analysis
9	Psychosocial aspects and patient self-help
10	Additional resources for health professionals and patients

Table 5: Preliminary table of contents before performing focus groups with the target group

The writing style was chosen such that health professionals with a certain degree of knowledge would feel addressed, but that it would still be comprehensible to read. While this kind of expert communication did not require a comparably thorough language level concept as for the patient brochures, overall comprehensibility of the brochure was examined in structured focus group interviews with physicians from gynaecological practices.

In addition to the writing style, the health professionals (e.g. gynaecologists and general practitioners that may not deal with hereditary breast and ovarian cancer on a day-to-day basis) were asked to provide feedback on the structure and contents, as well as layout and handling. Representatives from the patient organisation BRCA Netzwerk e.V. reviewed the brochures from the patient's point of view. The feedback gained is implemented in the brochures.

5 Experiences, Problems, and Lessons Learned

The key challenge of keeping information evidence-based and comprehensible was especially present in the brochures directed at patients, and even more for the Easy Language edition. To deal with this challenge, multiple editing loops were implemented, as shown in Figure 6 below. Included were several internal checks of content and language. Scientific accuracy was checked by in-house experts from CIS and CC-HBOC.

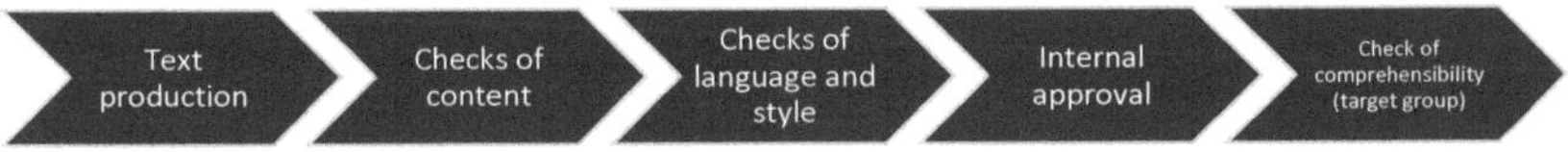

Figure 6: Simplified workflow for checks of Easy and Plain Language brochures.

Target group checks were conducted for the Easy Language brochure to test their comprehensibility. These checks are also an essential requirement for the production of Easy Language texts (Netzwerk Leichte Sprache 2021). For Plain Language materials, structured interviews are foreseen in order to retrieve feedback from the target groups, i.e. advice-seeking patients with hereditary cancer. These interviews will show whether the brochure concept meets the expectations of readers and which parts can be improved.

Limitations of Easy Language

Complex concepts concerning medical decisions

Although it is possible to provide information on cancer topics in Easy Language, there are some limitations as well. In order to translate health information into Easy Language, it is necessary to reduce the depth of information. In some cases, this may cause problems because the lack of certain in-depth information can make it difficult to use Easy Language materials to support medical decisions (Maaß/Rink 2020).

An example for that is the part on genetic testing in the Easy Language brochure on familial breast cancer. Whether or not a genetic test should be taken, is an individual decision. If someone sees a genetic test as beneficial or not is rather convoluted because it depends on the outcome. For example, if someone decides to take the test and the result is negative (meaning, there is no genetic predisposition), one might feel it was a good decision to take the test. On the other hand, if a test was taken and the result is positive (meaning, that there actually is a genetic predisposition and thus a higher cancer risk), individuals could feel they would rather not have known this. However, this depends a lot on a person's personal preferences and is thus difficult to explain in Easy Language. This might even result in emotional barriers that negatively influence text understanding of the recipients (Lang 2021: 131).

Resources

The production of Easy Language materials is quite resource-intensive as it takes not only time but also requires trained staff to produce Easy Language texts. As can be seen from the description of the editing process (see Figure 6), it binds staff resources for checks of content and language to ensure the quality of the information given. The obligatory target group checks and full illustration of the brochures need to be conducted externally, which generates additional costs to be considered.

Acceptance issues

As a very distinct form, Easy Language stands out from texts most people are used to. This results in a potential of stigmatisation of target groups (Zurstrassen 2015; Maaß 2020: 209).

Many people who could actually benefit from Easy Language might feel repulsed by such texts because of their unusual form that sometimes even has a "childish" look. One solution to this problem might be the use of other forms such as Easy Language Plus, a form that tries to combine the beneficial and accepted features of Easy Language and Plain Language (Maaß 2020).

However, from a survey that was conducted by CIS at the start of the familial breast and ovarian cancer project, it became evident that Easy Language Plus can also suffer from acceptance issues. Even though it has a standard text style, the sample text presented in the survey received mixed feedback (cf. Chapter 4.2 and Figure 4). While some readers appreciated the easy-to-read style, others stated it gave them the impression of being superficial. Although acceptance of such language forms might increase if they are more frequently used, it seems impossible to address all potential user groups with just one language level. Therefore, materials in different language levels and information depths are needed.

6 Conclusion and Perspectives

Despite the limitations of Easy Language (and in parts, of Plain Language as well), CIS has successfully transferred cancer-related health information into more comprehensible formats in order to reach target groups with low health literacy. Several materials on selected cancer topics were translated, laid out and illustrated in Easy Language.

Moreover, in a cooperation project dedicated to familial breast and ovarian cancer, CIS together with CC-HBOC developed brochures for patients and relatives in Easy Language and in Plain Language. These materials were developed alongside congruent information materials for physicians to tackle the challenge of low health literacy from both sides. Participation of the different target groups during the development process ensures that the user perspective is considered to optimise the materials.

However, at this point, the different brochures have so far not been evaluated in-depth, e.g., in intervention studies. It would be quite interesting to gain insights as to whether this approach is suitable to enhance health literacy and to support informed decision making, e.g., in the challenging context of hereditary cancer.

In the future, CIS aims to expand its portfolio by providing more easy-to-understand health information. Also, CIS intends to offer such texts not only in printed form, but also on its website.

Literature

Arbeitsgruppe GPGI 2016: "Gute Praxis Gesundheitsinformation / Good practice guidelines for health information". In: *Zeitschrift für Evidenz, Fortbildung und Qualität im Gesundheitswesen* 110–111, pp. 85–92.

Barber, Julia/Twelker, Maike/Wittenberg, Kerstin/Terfloth, Karin/Geulen, Julia/Weg-Remers, Susanne (2022): *Gute Tipps für ein kleineres Krebs·risiko*. Heidelberg: Krebsinformationsdienst.

BETZ, SABRINA/TERFLOTH, KARIN/KLEIN, STEFANIE/PENZKOFER, ANDREA/WEG-REMERS, SUSANNE (2017): *Lungen·krebs – was nun?* Heidelberg: Krebsinformationsdienst.

BREDEL, URSULA/MAAß, CHRISTIANE (2016): *Ratgeber Leichte Sprache*. Berlin: Duden.

DICK, JULIA/AUE, VIKTORIA/WESSELMANN, SIMONE/BRÉDART, ANNE/DOLBEAULT, SYLVIE/DEVILEE, PETER/STOPPA-LYONNET, DOMINIQUE/SCHMUTZLER, RITA K./RHIEM, KERSTIN (2021): "Survey on Physicians' Knowledge and Training Needs in Genetic Counseling in Germany." In: *Breast Care* 16 (4): pp. 389–395.

FADDA, MARTA/CHAPPUIS, PIERRE O./KATAPODI, MARIA C./PAGANI, OLIVIA/MONNERAT, CHRISTIAN/MEMBREZ, VÉRONIQUE/UNGER, SHEILA/ZUFFEREY, MARIA C. (2020): "Physicians communicating with women at genetic risk of breast and ovarian cancer: Are we in the middle of the ford between contradictory messages and unshared decision making?". In: *PLoS One* 15 (10): e0240054.

GIGERENZER, GERD/GAISSMAIER, WOLFGANG/KURZ-MILCKE, ELKE/SCHWARTZ, LISA M./WOLOSHIN, STEVEN (2017): "Helping Doctors and Patients Make Sense of Health Statistics." In: *Psychological Science in the Public Interest* 8 (2), pp. 53–96.

GROTLÜSCHEN, ANKE/BUDDEBERG, KLAUS/DUTZ, GREGOR/HEILMANN, LISANNE/STAMMER, CHRISTOPHER (2019): *LEO 2018 – Leben mit geringer Literalität*. Hamburg.

HANSEN-SCHIRRA, SILVIA/MAAß, CHRISTIANE (2020): "Easy Language, Plain Language, Easy Language Plus: Perspectives on Comprehensibility and Stigmatisation" In: HANSEN-SCHIRRA, SILVIA/MAAß, CHRISTIANE (eds.) (2020): *Easy language research: text and user perspectives*. Berlin: Frank & Timme, pp. 17–38.

HOWARD, A. FUCHSIA/BALNEAVES, LYNDA G./BOTTORFF, JOAN L. (2009): "Women's Decision Making about Risk-Reducing Strategies in the Context of Hereditary Breast and Ovarian Cancer: A Systematic Review." In: *Journal of Genetic Counseling* 18, pp. 578–597.

KELLERMANN, GUDRUN (2014): "Leichte und Einfache Sprache – Versuch einer Definition." (bpb, Hrsg.) In: *Aus Politik und Zeitgeschichte* (9-11/2014).

Klein, Stefanie/Geulen, Julia/Penzkofer, Andrea/Weg-Remers, Susanne/Terfloth, Karin (2020): "Lungen·krebs – Was nun? Eine Broschüre in Leichter Sprache." In: *PADUA* 15 (2), pp. 1–5.

Kuchenbaecker, Karoline B./Hopper, John L./Barnes, Daniel R./Phillips, Kelly-Anne/Mooij, Thea M./Roos-Blom, Marie-José/Jervis, Sarah/van Leeuwen, Flora E./Milne, Roger L./Andrieu, Nadine/Goldgar, David E./Terry, Mary B./Rookus, Matti A./Easton, Douglas F./Antoniou, Antonis C./BRCA1 and BRCA2 Cohort Consortium (2017): "Risks of Breast, Ovarian, and Contralateral Breast Cancer for BRCA1 and BRCA2 Mutation Carriers." In: *JAMA* 317 (23), pp. 2402–2416.

Lang, Katrin (2021): *Auffindbarkeit, Wahrnehmbarkeit, Akzeptabilität – Webseiten von Behörden in Leichter Sprache vor dem Hintergrund der rechtlichen Lage.* Berlin: Frank & Timme.

Lühnen, Julia/Albrecht, Martina/Mühlhauser, Ingrid/Steckelberg, Anke (2017): *Leitlinie evidenzbasierte Gesundheitsinformation.* Hamburg. https://www.leitlinie-gesundheitsinformation.de/

Maaß, Christiane (2015): *Leichte Sprache. Das Regelbuch.* Münster: LIT Verlag.

Maaß, Christiane/Rink, Isabel (2017): "Leichte Sprache: Verständlichkeit ermöglicht Gesundheitskompetenz." In: *Public Health Forum*, 25/1, pp. 50–53.

Maaß, Christiane (2020): *Easy Language – Plain Language – Easy Language Plus. Balancing Comprehensibility and Acceptability.* Berlin: Frank & Timme.

Maaß, Christiane/Rink, Isabel (2020): "Scenarios for Easy Language Translation: How to produce accessible content for users with diverse needs." In: Hansen-Schirra, Silvia/Maaß, Christiane (eds.): *Easy Language Research: Text and User Perspectives*. Berlin: Frank & Timme, pp. 41–56.

Nagler, Rebekah H./Yzer, Marco C./Rothman, Alexander J. (2019): "Effects of Media Exposure to Conflicting Information About Mammography: Results From a Population-based Survey Experiment." In: *Annals of Behavioural Medicine* 53 (10), pp. 896–908.

Netzwerk Leichte Sprache (2021): "Die Regeln für Leichte Sprache." https://www.leichte-sprache.org/leichte-sprache/die-regeln/ (accessed 2022-05-23)

Nippert, Irmgard/Julian-Reynier, Claire/Harris, Hilary/Evans, Gareth/van Asperen, Christi J./Tibben, Aad/Schmidtke, Jörg (2014): "Cancer risk communication, predictive testing and management in France, Germany, the Netherlands and the UK: general practitioners' and breast surgeons' current practice and preferred practice responsibilities." In: *Journal of Community Genetics* 5 (1), pp. 69–79.

Rocktäschel, Lucia C. (2020): "Gendern in Leichter Sprache – eine Anleitung." https://www.genderleicht.de/gendern-in-leichter-sprache-anleitung/ (accessed 2022-05-23).

Rosset, Magdalena/Reifegerste, Doreen/Baumann, Eva/Kludt, Evelyn/Weg-Remers, Susanne (2019): "Langzeittrends beim Krebsinformationsdienst (KID) des Deutschen Krebsforschungszentrums (DKFZ) Eine Analyse der Anfragen von Patientinnen und Patienten sowie Angehörigen von 1992 bis 2016." In: *Bundesgesundheitsblatt* 62, pp. 1120–1128.

Schaeffer, Doris/Berens, Eva-Maria/Gille, Svea/Griese, Lennert/Klinger, Julia/de Sombre, Steffen/Vogt, Dominique/Hurrelmann, Klaus (2021): *Gesundheitskompetenz der Bevölkerung in Deutschland – vor und während der Corona Pandemie: Ergebnisse des HLS-GER 2.* Bielefeld: Interdisziplinäres Zentrum für Gesundheitskompetenz-forschung (IZGK), Universität Bielefeld.

Schaeffer, Doris/Vogt, Dominique/Berens, Eva-Maria/Hurrelmann, Klaus (2016): *Gesundheitskompetenz der Bevölkerung in Deutschland.* Bielefeld.

Shaffer, Victoria A./Brodney, Suzanne/Gavaruzzi, Teresa/Zisman-Ilani, Yara/Munro, Sarah/Smith, Sian K./Thomas, Elizabeth/Valentine, Katherine D./Bekker, Hilary L. (2021): "Do Personal Stories Make Patient Decision Aids More Effective? An Update from the International Patient Decision Aids Standards." In: *Medical Decision Making* 41 (7), pp. 897–906.

Sørensen, Kristine/Van den Broucke, Stephan/Fullam, James/Doyle, Gerardine/Pelikan, Jürgen/Slonska, Zofia/Brand, Helmut (2012): "Health literacy and public health. A systematic review and integration of definitions and models." In: *BMC Public Health* 12: 80.

Winterbottom, Anna/Bekker, Hilary L./Conner, Mark/Mooney, Andrew (2008): "Does narrative information bias individual's decision making? A systematic review." In: *Social Science & Medicine* 67 (12), pp. 2079–2088.

Zurstrassen, Bettina (2015): "Inklusion durch Leichte Sprache? Eine kritische Einschätzung." In: *Didaktik der inklusiven politischen Bildung*, pp. 126–138.

Janine Michele / Martin Silke

Health literacy

Perspectives from occupational action of health care professionals

1 Initial problem

During their vocational training, health care professionals should acquire competencies that qualify them for their vocational actions. For these professions, the acquisition and communication of health literacy plays a key role.

For this reason, this article focuses on health literacy in the context of the vocational education of health care professionals. This group is highly heterogeneous within the German health care system and cannot be clearly defined (BMG 2021). In the following, health care professions are mainly understood as the so-called 'healing professions'. This occupational group is defined by the BMG as follows: 'The healing professions include those professions whose activities include the healing of diseases and the medical-assisting treatment and care of patients' (ibid.)[1]. Healing professions include, among others, the nursing professions, physiotherapy, ergotherapy, logopaedics and dietary assistance. The heterogenicity is mirrored not only in the various specific tasks and fields of work, but also in the vocational education in which the corresponding action competencies need to be developed.

The acquisition of the approbation and the use of the professional title is regulated by independent professional laws. These also include the training and examination regulations and set a mandatory framework for the organization of vocational training. The differentiation between the professional laws var-

1 Quote translated by authors. Original published version: "Zu den Heilberufen zählen diejenigen Berufe, deren Tätigkeit die Heilung von Krankheiten und die medizinisch-helfende Behandlung und Betreuung von Patienten erfasst" (BMG 2021).

ies tremendously. However, none of the training and examination regulations of the professions mentioned explicitly address the term health literacy (cf. PflAPrV 2018; ErgThAPrV 1999; PhysTh-APrV 1994; LogAPrO 1980; DiätAss-APrV 1994). Health literacy can therefore be defined as the cognitive, social and motivational abilities and skills of an individual that contribute to independently accessing health-related information and being able to understand and apply it in a way that promotes disease management, disease prevention and/or health promotion (cf. Dierks 2017: 2; Bitzer/Sørensen 2018: 754). Discussing the topic of health literacy in the context of occupational action of health professions is relevant under two different perspectives: On the one hand, health care professionals are considered to fulfil a significant role in promoting the health literacy of their patients (Schaeffer et al. 2020; Kolpatzik/Schaeffer/Vogt 2018: 84f.). On the other hand, the individual health literacy of the professionals themselves can contribute to the maintenance of their own health in the context of occupational action and beyond. For both angles, accessible communication is a major requirement. The key to achieving such accessibility is the adaptation of communication offers for the intended aims and target groups (cf. Maaß/Rink 2018: 20). To promote the health literacy of their patients, health care professionals must have the ability to identify and overcome different barriers to offer health-related information in a comprehensible form. Similarly to promoting health care professionals' own health literacy, teachers and trainers must take a communicative approach that addresses all of the students' needs. During their vocational qualification, students therefore need to be taught two different aspects of the field of health literacy. Both are related to their vocational action competence in different ways.

In vocational education, action orientation as a theoretical learning principle is the basis for curriculum development and methodological-didactic approaches (KMK 2021: 17). In following, the didactic principle of action orientation will be discussed. In doing so, the potential of action-oriented teaching-learning concepts is discussed with regards to the acquisition of individual health literacy of health care professionals, as well as with regards to the competencies required to promote the health literacy of patients. Using the concept of vocational action competence, aspects of the vocational action of health professionals will be contextualized in connection with the mentioned perspectives on the topic of health literacy. Since health literacy of individuals always needs to be considered in interaction with their surroundings, an outlook on the consequences for health-promoting environments and the implications regarding organizational health literacy will be given in this context.

2 Vocational action competence and action orientation in vocational training

One aim of the present article is to analyse current understandings and guidelines about the orientation of didactic action regarding their transferability to concepts for the promotion of health literacy on the two levels outlined above. Thereby, we address the corresponding problem of the classification of health competence for health care professionals in the framework of their occupational activities. In 2005, the guiding principle of vocational action competence was anchored in § 1 of the Vocational Training Act (BBiG). Thus, an approach was legally enshrined that aims not only to impart content and knowledge, but also to focus on the interlinking of knowledge and action, of reflection and action (cf. Euler 2020: 206). In the following, the underlying theoretical construct of professional action competence will be explained and the extent to which action orientation can help in the preparation of didactic curricular content will be presented.

Afterwards, in Chapter 3, a proposal for the accessible, action-oriented teaching of health literacy in vocational pedagogical settings will be made on this basis.

2.1 Vocational action competence

Action competence describes the potential of a person to act (at least in the medium term) in similar types of situations. Vocational action competence is "[…] the ability and willingness to act in a professionally, personally and socially competent manner in work-related situations and to further develop one's ability to act in accordance with one's vocational and social responsibility"

(Dehnbostel)[2]. The Standing Conference of the Ministers of Education and Cultural Affairs of the Federal Republic of Germany (Kultusministerkonferenz) also formulated the aim of vocational education and training as, among other things, enabling the acquisition of cross-occupational and work-related competencies to enable people to practice their occupation and help shape society. Accordingly, particular emphasis is placed on vocational action competence.

Therefore, students are expected to behave in a situation-appropriate and properly thought-out manner in future professional and private actions and to act in an individually and socially responsible manner (cf. KMK 2018: 2). This refocused the goals of vocational education and training in line with the labour market. The input-oriented direction of educational and learning processes gave way to an outcome orientation in the conception and design of vocational education (cf. Gillen 2013: 1). Vocational action competence is divided into methodological, technical, social and human competence to qualify learners beyond the content of a vocational profile and to enable them to engage in lifelong learning. This requires that vocational school teaching be designed by teachers who operate in a dual role. They are simultaneously experts in their profession with technical knowledge and competence, as well as pedagogues with the task of offering diverse competence promotion from their repertoire (cf. Meyer 2020: 555). The core of their pedagogical work is therefore the promotion or respectively the acquisition of vocational action competence as a goal of vocational education (cf. KMK 2018: 11). Within this framework, it is therefore necessary to develop competencies for specific, primarily vocational contexts of action and scenarios that are situated out of their realistic context. The construction leads from the (professional) situation via the required performance to the knowledge that is demanded and expressed in this performance (cf. Gillen 2013: 1). The vocational educational understanding of competence therefore suggests taking vocational action situations as the starting point of the conception of teaching-learning processes. The

2 Quote translated by authors. Original published version: "[...] die Fähigkeit und Bereitschaft, in beruflichen Situationen fach-, personal- und sozialkompetent zu handeln und seine Handlungsfähigkeit in beruflicher und gesellschaftlicher Verantwortung weiterzuentwickeln" (Dehnbostel 2015: p. 19).

curricular transfer thus follows a guiding principle that is oriented towards a corresponding complete action.

2.2 Action orientation as a didactic-curricular guideline

Vocational education aims at enabling people to occupational action. Teaching-learning approaches, such as the "Intimatio principle" which is based on demonstrating and imitating occupational action, can already be found in the medieval times of the guilds (cf. Herkner/Pahl 2020: 190). At the level of educational policy and research, the action-orientation approach forms the overcoming of the learning-centred dualism between thinking and acting (ibid; Czycholl 2009: 173). In delineation to the teaching of systematic factual knowledge, it represents a reformed approach in vocational education since the work-orientated turn (Rommel/Michele 2019: 30; Eckert 1992: 59). Even if action orientation is aimed at the occupation-like structures and the transmission of vocational action knowledge, it has been primarily located in the context of vocational schools for about thirty years (see Pätzold 1992). This was established in the 1990s by the reorganization of apprenticeships, including the introduction of the learning field concept by the Standing Conference of the Ministers of Education and Cultural Affairs of the Federal Republic of Germany as a benchmark for curriculum development. According to the didactic principles (KMK 2021: 17), the emphasis on action orientation should also enable young people to plan, carry out and reflect on work tasks independently. (ibid; Herkner/Pahl 2020: 193). Following this procedural approach, the didactic principles on learning situations, which are derived from concrete professional actions (KMK 2021: 17f.) are:

- When planning and executing action-oriented teaching from the perspective of learning theory and didactics, the following points of reference can be pointed out:
- Didactic points of reference are situations that are significant for occupational practice.
- Learning takes place in complete actions, as far as possible performed by the students themselves or at least logically followed by them.

- Actions enhance the holistic understanding of professional reality in an increasingly globalized and digitalized world of life and work (e.g., economic, ecological, legal, technical, safety-related, professional, technical and foreign-language, social and ethical aspects).
- Actions refer to the experiences of the learners.
- Actions integrate social processes, for example, the declaration of interests or the management of conflicts, as well as different perspectives on career and life planning. (ibid.)

While breaking up and interlinking subject- and action-systematic teaching structures, a completely new demand was placed on the methodological-didactic framework. (Hacker/Skell 1993: 268ff.). The process of a complete action, which consists of six elements, strives for holistic learning through the connection of thinking and acting. Such actions are considered complete because actions involve thinking as well as practical activities and affective attitudes (Bonz 1999; Hacker/Skell 1993: 268ff.). The essential characteristic of the steps of a 'complete professional action' is the connection of thinking and acting processes, which due to its processual character, emphasizes the concrete meaning of the contents for the professions. This problem orientation ensures a high degree of openness, which allows a wide scope for the development of professional, social, personal and methodical competencies. Another key element is the students' participation in planning and formulating the learning targets of the courses. In this way, motivation and identification with the lessons can be ensured. The learning process that builds on this takes place in complete actions that are holistically oriented to and determined by the actions of the students. For this purpose, it is necessary to go through various individual steps, each of which serves its own purpose in the circular process (KMK 1997: 27; Herkner/Pahl 2020: 193).

1. Informing: The learner should independently obtain an overview of the situation to identify the steps required to collect and sort necessary information.
2. Planning: Several possibilities that are suitable for the situation have to be worked out and compared with each other.

3. Deciding: Possibilities are finally contrasted and decided upon, either alone or in collaboration
4. Executing: The learner executes the required work steps as independently as possible.
5. Controlling: The subject of learning should be checked by the learner as independently as possible. This includes addressing issues such as the correct processing of the assignment and the targets to be achieved.
6. Evaluating: The entire vocational action is always completed by reflecting on the whole work process. In this process, the learner becomes aware of his or her actions and learning successes so that the outcome does not remain accidental. (Konrad 2017: 196; Rommel/Michele 2019: 31).

It should be noted that the characteristics of the complete action, do not have to be in a stringent order. Individual steps can be repeated or exchanged when needed, depending on how it is most conducive to the process. Originally transferred from work science to vocational education, it is possible to differentiate vocational actions and adapt them to the competence and knowledge level of the learners.

Building on the concept of complete action, the framework curricula of vocational schools have been structured according to the learning field concept since the mid-1990s (KMK 2018: 2). Oriented to vocational actions, these learning fields build on each other in their complexity and integrate sub-disciplines into the vocational action. In this way, the learning situations become more complex, but also holistic, so for example, health-related information is not – out of context as in the above-mentioned subject system – but is integrated into all other sub-disciplines. The complete vocational action can thus be taught with all sub-disciplines in a goal-oriented and application-related manner, whereby the learners always identify with the action due to their involvement and learn actively (cf. Schelten 2010: 187).

Focusing on the target group of this contribution, the following chapter will consider the extent to which action orientation is suitable as a basic concept for preparing and conveying occupation-specific content. Special attention is drawn to the role of health literacy within the occupational profile itself and – in contrast to this – to the health literacy that is to be imparted to the individuals themselves. In order to put these in relation to each other, the guiding principle of vocational training, vocational action competence, is used as an orientation (cf. Dehnbostel 2015: 17). Nevertheless, it must be taken into account that VET institutions can also always form a framework to enable and promote health literacy and health literate behaviour. In this way, they can also contribute to the promotion of accessibility at the organizational level.

3 Health literacy teaching in vocational education

From the very first results on the health literacy of the population in Germany (cf. Schaeffer/Berens/Vogt 2017), the question arose of how to improve the health literacy of the population. This resulted, among other things, in the National Action Plan Health Literacy with relevant recommendations to strengthen the health literacy of the people (cf. Schaeffer/Hurrelmann/Bauer/Kolpatzik 2020). The plan describes the promotion of health literacy as a task for society, but also emphasizes the importance of health professionals, who can and should take a key role, particularly in disease management (ibid.: 48f.). Findings from the follow-up survey put yet more emphasis on the demands and recommendations: while the percentage of people with limited health literacy in the initial survey from 2016 was at 54.3 %. The 2020 survey showed an increase to 58.8 % (cf. Schaeffer/Berens/Vogt 2017; Schaeffer et al. 2021). The promotion of health literacy is only slowly being recognized as a task in the healthcare professions.

Thus, Kolpatzik, Schaeffer and Vogt (2018: 75ff.) describe the promotion of health literacy as a task of nursing in the context of the "Agenda Pflege 2021", but also state the lack of presence of the topic in the care sector, the insufficient qualification of health professionals in the promotion of health literacy, as well as a lack of implementation in curricula of vocational education, training and further education (ibid.: 85). The situation is similar in the therapeutic professions: In physiotherapy, a nationwide stocktaking on the construct health literacy showed that about 40 % of the interviewed therapists are unfamiliar with the term health literacy (cf. Wirner et al. 2020). At the same time, the participants estimated the role of physiotherapy in the promotion of health literacy as high to very high at more than 70 % (ibid.).

Although the German Association of Occupational Therapy has included the promotion of health literacy in the competence profile of ergotherapy, the topic is not included in mandatory curricula in this sector. It can therefore not be assumed that members of the profession are specifically taught the necessary competencies during their training, to deal with a possibly low level of health literacy or to promote health literacy. This circumstance could also be a reason why the health care professions do not yet fully recognize and endorse the task of promoting the health literacy of their patients as such. Although there are already sources of materials and methods for measuring and promoting the health literacy of patients (cf. Schmidt-Kaehler et al. 2017), there is still a lack of integration into a concrete educational concept (cf. Kolpatzik/Schaeffer/Vogt 2018: 85f.).

At this point, the concept of action orientation described in the previous chapter offers an important orientation for the development of educational concepts and the promotion of health literacy by members of the health care professions.

When the goal-oriented promotion of a patient's health literacy is understood as a task of the health care professions, the competencies required for this are to be seen as part of the vocational action competence of the respective health care professions. The competence requirements that the performance of the occupation demands is usually derived from the description of the respective occupational field of action, which is characterized by related situations of action and associated tasks (cf. Klemme 2012: 184). The description of typical occupational situations can exemplify the challenges posed by the aim of promoting patient's health literacy for the competencies of health care professionals. The following situation may serve as an example to describe the competence requirements:

> *A physiotherapist has been treating a patient diagnosed with a herniated disc for a few days. The patient had experienced a sudden stabbing pain in his back a few weeks ago when he was lifting a heavy object. After the*

pain would not subside even days later and began radiating into the right leg, an MRI of the lumbar spine was conducted. The findings showed a herniated disc. In response, the doctor prescribed physiotherapy and the patient started an out-patient physiotherapeutic treatment. Now the patient is very distressed and still has slight pain.

In such a situation, patients encounter many challenges. Bitzer/Sørensen (2018: 755) characterize an individual's health literacy as a dynamic and context-bound concept that requires an adaptation of existing competencies or, if necessary, the acquisition of new competencies when changes occur. The appearance of the health problem described in the current case represented a change in context, which required the patient to adapt his or her individual health literacy.

Promoting this individual health literacy, adapted to the new context, can be understood as the therapist's task. If one considers vocational action competence in its subdivision into technical, methodological, social and human competence, the promotion of the patient's individual health literacy by the therapist requires skills in all dimensions. Thus, health care professionals need appropriate expertise in the construct of health literacy, its characteristics and its significance for the health of patients. On the level of methodical competence, tools and strategies are required to be able to measure and promote the health literacy of patients. Here, the material and method collections previously referred to can be checked for applicability in the respective professional context and then integrated into education, training and further education. Social competence in this context primarily relates to communication aspects. In situations such as those described above, health care professionals must be able to recognize and overcome communication barriers in order to communicate health-related information in an accessible and patient-specific way. On this basis, they can fulfil a key role in creating access to health information. For this purpose, it is important to incorporate evidence from health communication research. In this context, Baumann (2018: 27f.) emphasizes the importance of optimizing not only the quality of content, but also the quality of communication, and criticizes the generally too narrow understanding of communication of information in the health care system: "To put it bluntly, however, an oversimplified model of information communication is often used as a basis, which essentially assumes that information can be administered to patients as with a subcutaneous injection. Thus, it is often neglected that health-related decisions – even more so in the case of acute affection – are usually not made rationally. The search for, but also the avoidance of, health information takes place based on one's own or vicarious prior experience, emotionally determined attitudes, perceptions and expectations of competence, and is influenced by perceptions of insecurity and the need for assistance, as well as by the social environment"[3] (ibid.).

The description illustrates the great complexity of communicating health-related information and hence the high demands placed on social competence and the associated ability of health care professionals to communicate without barriers, which cannot be achieved solely by avoiding technical terms. It also becomes clear that the defined areas of competence cannot be viewed separately from one another. Rather, technical, social and personal aspects are interdependent and systemically interlinked (cf. Schröder 2004: 199).

Kolpatzik, Schaeffer and Vogt state that educational tasks with a communicative or information and knowledge transfer character play a subordinate role in the curricula of education, training and continuing education in nursing (cf. ibid. 2018: 85). Promoting these competencies in the education and training of health care professionals and integrating them into the corresponding curricula will be an important task of vocational education in the health care professions in the future.

To reflect and critically question the handling of patients with possibly low health literacy or the promotion of health literacy in one's own professional actions is based on human competence as part of the vocational action competence of health care professionals. This underlines once again that addressing

3 Quote translated by authors. Original published version: "Zugespitzt formuliert wird jedoch häufiger ein zu einfaches Modell der Informationsvermittlung zugrunde gelegt, das im Kern davon ausgeht, den Patienten Informationen wie mit einer subkutanen Injektion verabreichen zu können. So wird häufig vernachlässigt, dass gesundheitsrelevante Entscheidungen – erst recht im Falle einer akuten Betroffenheit – meist nicht rational getroffen werden. Die Suche nach, aber auch die Vermeidung von Gesundheitsinformationen erfolgt auf Basis eigener oder stellvertretender Vorerfahrungen, emotional geprägter Einstellungen, Vorstellungen und Kompetenzerwartungen und wird von Unsicherheitswahrnehmungen und Unterstützungsbedarfen sowie vom sozialen Umfeld beeinflusst" (Baumann 2018: 27f).

the issue of health literacy is the basis for health care professionals recognizing the promotion of health literacy as their task in the first place.

4 Health literacy as part of one's own vocational action competence

As already mentioned, the health literacy of health care professionals has a twofold importance for their professional education. On the one hand, they must develop their own health literacy, and on the other hand, they must be able to improve the health literacy of their patients as part of their occupational practice. Following this differentiation, the question now arises as to how this distinction affects the design of vocational qualification in order to fulfil this requirement.

For this purpose, the described model of vocational action competence is used to analyse the extent to which the competence profiles can be classified in this model and what this means in the context of accessibility in the acquisition of health literacy.

The practical example of action-oriented teaching for health care professionals already shows the interdependence of the competence dimensions addressed. The training of social, technical and human competencies is based on the one hand on the work-related and on the other hand on the individual parameters of health literacy. For the target group, it is now necessary to establish an awareness of – and relationship between – the two scopes of health literacy within the framework of their vocational education. This transition can now succeed through the process of reflection. Thus, learning alongside the complete action succeeds above all based on its reflection (KMK 1997: 27) and is thus an integral component in the context of the educational process. Here, therefore, a targeted differentiation can take place. The abstraction of experience in the reflection process does not focus on the bare generation of knowledge, but lies in reinterpreting experiences of action, developing concrete problem-solving strategies, questioning previous beliefs and testing them in renewed action (Roters 2012; Busse 2021: 11).

The professional actions of health care professionals are not only relevant in terms of their role in promoting the health literacy of their patients; rather, it is also the health literacy of health care professional themselves that is of central importance given the health-related burdens of practicing in these professions. The relatively high health burden compared to others is most evident in the nursing profession. Demographic change with an increasing number of people in need of care (cf. Federal Statistical Office 2018) and a simultaneous shortage of skilled workers leads to stressful work demands such as time and performance pressure (cf. Mojtahedzadeh et al. 2021: 16). In addition, there is usually heavy physical work with people in need of care, the work organization in the shift system, as well as psychologically stressful situations. The high level of stress is also expressed in the above-average number of days of incapacity to work among employees in this sector (cf. Techniker Krankenkasse 2019: 28). Added to this are the major physical and psychological strains (ibid.: 65). Besides the aforementioned conditions in the field of work that are detrimental to health, initial empirical studies on the health behaviour of nursing staff also reveal an unhealthy diet, a deficit of physical activity, or a lack of opportunities for breaks and regeneration units (cf. Mojtahedzadeh et al. 2021: 18). The National Action Plan Health Literacy also focuses on the education system, as well as the professional and working field in its recommendations (cf. Schaeffer, et al. 2020: 31). Given the health burdens described in the example of nursing, health professionals should not only be enabled to promote the health literacy of their patients but should also be strengthened in their own health literacy. Vocational training institutions should specifically strengthen the health literacy of future health care professionals. In addition, the professional group of teachers is itself particularly at high risk for chronic stress and the development of mental illnesses due to their occupational framework (cf. Albrecht 2016: 11). Having the necessary knowledge, skills and abilities to make health-promoting decisions in the context of one's own professional activities, i.e., to act in a health-competent manner in the professional context, should be understood as part of professional action competence and promoted accordingly in the context of education, training and continuing education. There is an increasing shift of perspective in the discourse on health literacy. It is not the individual alone who bears the responsibility, but institutions and social systems should also create a framework which their users can easily navigate and in which resources are offered in a way that is appropriate to the target group to facilitate health-promoting decisions (cf. Schaefer/Bitzer/Dierks 2019: 5). This task should be performed by institutions in which people are confronted with health issues or decisions (cf. ibid.: 3). Accordingly, health care institutions and the actors operating in these institutions are of major importance. Accordingly, health care institutions and the female actors operating in these institutions are of the utmost importance. When considering health literacy at the organizational level, two central questions arise: First, the health burdens in the nursing field were described at the beginning of this chapter. Is it possible to promote health literacy in an institution if this is also an environment in which the people are confronted with working conditions that are highly detrimental to their health? On the other hand, can health care professionals effectively promote the health literacy of their patients at all if the facilities they work for provide a low organizational health literacy for their users?

5 Conclusion

Given the above, this paper has presented different perspectives on health literacy from the health care professionals' point of view. Here, it has been shown that the construct of health literacy is tangential to the professional actions of health care professionals in several ways. The central role that health care professionals can and should play in the future in promoting the health literacy of their patients is a perspective that was illustrated and in the context of which the empowerment of health care professionals to communicate without barriers is indispensable. Focusing on the health care professionals' own individual health literacy, which is necessary in order to be able to make health-promoting decisions in a field of work characterized by high physical and psychological stress, represents a central approach. To this end, it makes sense to involve the experts of the respective health care professions working in the facilities in such issues. Health care professionals are often in a position to identify barriers at the organizational or systemic level and to help initiate appropriate improvements. Designing health-competent organizations by decision-makers far from patients does, in itself, not appear to be useful. However, the health care professions must also recognize and acknowledge the design of health-competent organizations as a task. Likewise, health professions must design their own working environment in a way that is conducive to health.

Accessible communication between teachers and learners is a prerequisite for promoting health literacy among future health professionals and is tied to teachers' abilities to communicate appropriately.

In addition, future tasks of health care professionals in the design of health literacy-promoting organizations were outlined. Acquiring all these competencies related to the construct of health literacy is not least the task of the vocational education and training institutions of the respective health care professions.

The model of vocational action competence and the associated outcome orientation in vocational education (cf. Gillen 2013: 4) offers the opportunity to anchor health literacy in the training of health care professionals. With the concept of action orientation as a guideline for the curricular-methodological transfer of vocational education, approaches to solutions could be shown in the respective perspectives. In order to be able to meet the diverse requirements in the context of the topic in the future, the various professions must derive appropriate competencies based on occupational action situations and promote their development in the learners. In this way, health literacy can be sensitized and promoted among health care professionals in their various areas of application within the framework of their professional action.

Literature

Baumann, Eva (2018): "Gesundheitskompetenz als Kommunikationsherausforderung". In: *GGW* 18, pp. 23–30.

Bitzer, Eva-M./Sørensen, Kristine (2018): "Gesundheitskompetenz-Health Literacy". In: *Das Gesundheitswesen* 80, pp. 754–766.

BMG (2021): "*Gesundheitsberufe: eine Übersicht*" Online: https://www.bundesgesundheitsministerium.de/themen/gesundheitswesen/gesundheitsberufe/gesundheitsberufe-allgemein.html (last accessed: 18.8.2021).

Bonz, Bernhard (1999): *Methoden der Berufsbildung. Ein Lehrbuch*. Stuttgart: Hirzel Verlag.

Pätzold, G. (1992): *Handlungsorientierung in der beruflichen Bildung.* Frankfurt a. M.: Gesellschaft zur Förderung arbeitsorientierter Forschung und Bildung.

PflAPrV (2018): "*Ausbildungs- und Prüfungsverordnung für die Pflegeberufe*". Online: https://www.gesetzeiminternet.de/pflaprv/.pdf (last accessed: 18.8.2021).

PhysTh-APrV (1994): "*Ausbildungs- und Prüfungsverordnung für Physiotherapeuten*". Online: https://www.gesetze-im-internet.de/physthaprv/PhysThAPrV.pdf (last accessed: 18.8.2021).

Roters, Bianca (2012): *Professionalisierung durch Reflexion in der Lehrerbildung.* Münster, Waxmann.

Rommel, Irina/Michele, Janine (2020): Educational Guidelines and Didactical Principles in Germans TVET-System: Skilling through Complete Vocational Action, In: *Journal of Engineering, Science & Management Education*, 13 (1), pp. 28–32.

Schaeffer, Doris/Berens, Eva M./Vogt, Dominique (2017): "Gesundheitskompetenz der Bevölkerung in Deutschland – Ergebnisse einer repräsentativen Befragung". In: *Deutsches Ärzteblatt* 114 (4), pp. 53–60.

Schaeffer, Doris/Berens, Eva M./Gille, Svea/Griese, Lennert/Klinger, Julia/de Sombre, Steffen/Vogt, Dominique/Hurrelmann, Klaus (2021): Gesundheitskompetenz der Bevölkerung in Deutschland – vor und während der Corona Pandemie: *Ergebnisse des HLS GER 2.* Bielefeld: Interdisziplinäres Zentrum für Gesundheitskompetenzforschung (IZGK).

Schaefer, Corinna/Bitzer, Eva M./Dierks, Marie L. für den Vorstand des DNGK (2019): "*Mehr Organisationale Gesundheitskompetenz in die Gesundheitsversorgung bringen! Ein Positionspapier des DNGK*". Online: https://dngk.de/wp-content/uploads/2019/11/DNGK-PosPap-OGK-final_19115.pdf (l last accessed: 31.8.2021).

Schaeffer, Doris/Hurrelmann, Klaus/Bauer, Ullrich/Kolpatzik, Kai (eds.): (2020): Nationaler Aktionsplan Gesundheitskompetenz: Die Gesundheitskompetenz in Deutschland stärken (1. überarbeitete Auflage). Berlin: KomPart.

Schelten, Andreas (2010): "Einführung in die Berufspädagogik". In: Petzold, Georg (ed.): *Handlungsorientierung in der beruflichen Bildung.* Frankfurt a. M.: Stuttgart. Gesellschaft zur Förderung arbeitsorientierter Forschung und Bildung, pp. 55–78.

Schmidt-Kaehler, Sebastian/Vogt, Dominique/Berens, Eva M./Schaeffer, Doris (2017): *"Gesundheitskompetenz: Verständlich informieren und beraten. Material- und Methodensammlung zur Verbraucher- und Patientenberatung für Zielgruppen mit geringer Gesundheitskompetenz"*. Online: https://www.uni-bielefeld.de/gesundhw/ag6/downloads/Material_und_Methodensammlung.pdf (last accessed: 18.8.2021).

Sekretariat der Kultusministerkonferenz – (KMK) (2021): *Handreichungen für die Erarbeitung von Rahmenlehrplänen der Kultusministerkonferenz für den berufsbezogenen Unterricht in der Berufsschule und ihre Abstimmung mit Ausbildungsordnungen des Bundes für anerkannte Ausbildungsberufe*. Bonn. Online: https://www.kmk.org/fileadmin/veroeffentlichungen_beschluesse/2021/2021_06_17-GEP-Handreichung.pdf (last accessed: 01.09.2021).

Sekretariat der Kultusministerkonferenz – (KMK) (2018): *Handreichung für die Erarbeitung von Rahmenlehrplänen der Kultusministerkonferenz für den berufsbezogenen Unterricht in der Berufsschule und ihre Abstimmung mit Ausbildungsordnungen des Bundes für anerkannte Ausbildungsberufe*. Berlin. Online: https://www.kmk.org/fileadmin/Dateien/veroeffentlichungen_beschluesse/2011/2011_09_23-GEP-Handreichung.pdf (last accessed: 18.8.2021).

Sekretariat der Kultusministerkonferenz – (KMK) (1997): *Handreichungen für die Erarbeitung von Rahmenlehrplänen der Kultusminister- konferenz für den berufsbezogenen Unterricht in der Berufsschule und ihre Abstimmung mit Ausbildungsordnungen des Bundes für anerkannte Ausbildungsberufe*. Bonn Beschluss vom 12.06.1997.

Sekretariat der Kultusministerkonferenz – (KMK) (1991): *Rahmenvereinbarung über die Berufsschule*. Beschluss der Kultusministerkonferenz vom 15.03.1991. Bonn. Online: https://www.kmk.org/fileadmin/Dateien/pdf/PresseUndAktuelles/Beschluesse_Veroeffentlichungen/rvbs91-03-15.pdf (last accessed: 18.8.2021).

Statistisches Bundesamt (2018): "*Pflegestatistik – Pflege im Rahmen der Pflegeversicherung: Deutschlandergebnisse*" Online: https://www.destatis.de/DE/Themen/Gesellschaft-Umwelt/Gesundheit/Pflege/_inhalt.html (last accessed: 18.8.2021).

Wirner, Corinna/Pott, Claudia/Kirschneck, Michaela/Coenen, Michaela (2020): "Bundesweite Bestandsaufnahme zum Konstrukt Gesundheitskompetenz aus der Perspektive der Profession Physiotherapie. In: *Das Gesundheitswesen*. Stuttgart/New York: Georg Thieme Verlag, pp. 60–63.

Giulia Pedrini

Diathesis in comprehensibility-enhanced texts in the medical field

An analysis of layperson summaries of clinical trials

1 Introduction

Accessibility in the medical field has been gaining increasing importance in the last decades. While terminology in specialised texts is the most evident source of issues for non-experts, other linguistic features undoubtedly contribute to text complexity. One of these is diathesis, which will be analysed in a medical text type ascribable to the Plain Language variant, i.e. layperson summaries of clinical trial results.

1.1 Diathesis and active-passive opposition in English and German

Diatheses are defined as grammatical verb conditions such as active, passive, antipassive, middle, reflexive, causative, or applicative (Wunderlich 1993: 730). It goes without saying that not all of these play a major role in every language; for instance, the antipassive diathesis is a characteristic studied primarily in ergative languages, such as Basque (Leiss 1992: 88–96; Cooreman 1994: 50). For the purposes of this paper a suitable definition is provided by Shibatani (1988: 3), according to whom "voice[1] is to be understood as a mechanism that selects a grammatically prominent syntactic constituent – subject – from the underlying semantic functions (case or thematic roles) of a clause". Similarly,

1 As will be indicated by the next definition, "voice" is a synonym of "diathesis". Another synonymous term, more frequently used in German-speaking literature, is *genus verbi*.

König and Gast (2009: 122) state that "the term 'voice' (or 'diathesis') relates to the argument structure of predicates, i.e. the relationship between thematic roles like Agent, Patient, Instrument and grammatical functions like subject and object, as well as to the alternations found between different argument structures".

As the authors (ibid.: 123) point out, the main voice opposition in German and English, found in traditional descriptions, is active-passive. They also state that the basic diathesis is provided by the active voice. Likewise, Shibatani (1988: 3), discussing accusative languages and therefore indirectly also English and German, points out that the basic strategy for these languages consists in selecting an agent for the subject role, and that the resulting unmarked structure is the active voice, whereas the passive voice is marked. Also, Chomsky (1957), in his transformational-generative grammar (TGG), derives passive sentences from active ones. In their Relational Grammar (RG), an alternative to TGG, Perlmutter and Postal (1983) state that all verbs have several strata of potential syntactic projections ("diatheses") and changes[2] that may occur between them. According to this theory, each stratum implies only the relations 1 (subject), 2 (direct object) and 3 (indirect object), as well as potential obliques. In passivisation, a constituent with a lower status in the relational hierarchy may be promoted or advanced. This, in turn, leads to the demotion of another constituent due to the stratal uniqueness law, which does not allow the presence of two arguments for the same function (Wunderlich 1993: 735–736).

The prototypical passive forms in English and German are BE + PAST PARTICIPLE and WERDEN (*Vorgangspassiv*) or SEIN (*Zustandspassiv*)[3] + PAST PARTICIPLE, respectively. Beside these traditional forms, more and more researchers are also focusing on alternative structures which may be subsumed under the category of passivity from a semantic (although not always syntactic) point of

2 Terms referring to derivations from the active voice which may be found in literature are "valency change" (or "changing"), "relation change", "argument shifting", and "grammatical function changing" (cf. *inter alia* Wunderlich [1993: 730]).

3 It should be noted that, according to some linguists (e.g. Alexiadou/Schäfer 2013: 1–2), *Zustandspassiv* is not canonical due to its auxiliary. Leiss (1992: 156–186) goes so far as to situate it between passive and aspect as a resultative.

view (cf. e.g. Lenz 2006). An overview of these passive-related structures will be provided later in the paper (2.2).

1.2 Passive diathesis in Languages for Specific Purposes

While studies concerning Languages for Specific Purposes (LSPs) were initially limited to terminology and phraseology research, in the last decades they have embraced other aspects, too, such as morphosyntax. Nowadays it is widely recognised that technical terms are not the only features of specialised language. However, whereas each LSP is characterised by the presence of its own dominion of technical terms, its morphosyntactic features do not substantially differ from those of general language; what does indeed vary is the frequency of such features as well as their functions (cf. e.g. Scarpa 2008: 40). In this respect, Halliday (1990: 57–58) goes as far as to talk about "a typical syndrome of grammatical features" in LSPs for their increased frequency compared to general language. These morphosyntactic features entail passivisation, nominalisation as well as information condensation. Clearly, in this paper I will focus on the former.

As has been highlighted, the passive diathesis is more frequent in LSPs (in written texts or oral discourse with characteristics of written text types, such as presentations) than in general language. However, this increased frequency is only relative, as the active diathesis still remains more frequent than the passive one in absolute terms within LSPs, too (cf. e.g. Roelcke 1999: 77; Magris 1992: 70). In a corpus analysis regarding diathesis conducted on a wide range of text types, Svartvik (1966: 164–165) found that even in the subcorpus with the highest occurrence of passive forms, i.e. "scientific exposition", the proportion of passives to actives was not higher than 1:3. Similarly, in Sager et al. (1980: 209) the passive diathesis of technical-scientific texts is compared to that of literary prose, resulting in a percentage ranging from 26 to 32.6 % for the former, and a strikingly – although not surprisingly – low 2.2–3 % for the latter.

Many explanations are provided by scholars and linguists for this increased frequency. Magris (1992: 70) states that passive forms allow information to be provided in a neutral way, i.e. not highlighting the agent – which is often even omitted – but the action itself. Agent omission is discussed also, among others, by König and Gast (2009: 123), who point out that agents are often omitted if they are not considered to be relevant or are not easily specifiable. This is connected to a tendency towards anonymisation and objectivisation, paramount in specialised discourse. Finally, another frequent explanation in literature is that the passive diathesis impacts on LSP theme-rheme progression.

1.3 Passive diathesis, comprehensibility, and text simplification

In spite of its functions and role in LSPs, the passive diathesis is generally said to be more difficult than the active one, as it implies a higher cognitive load for readers. Evidence of this complexity is provided also by its relative late acquisition in children, shown among others by experiments conducted by Grimm (1975). Likewise, Lenz (2006: 75) states that this phenomenon is particularly difficult to acquire for foreign language learners. Bredel and Maaß (2016: 313–314), referring to the German language, attribute the complexity of the passive diathesis to two main factors: firstly, a semantic reason, since the event representation is more abstract than in active sentences. The agent must be inferred, as it does not appear in the surface structure. In this respect, Maaß (2015: 78–80), in the context of German Easy Language, stated that action orientation is one of the main principles for text simplification, and agents should be explicit to clarify who is performing an action[4]. However, according to Duden (2016: 561), agents are predominantly omitted (in approximately 90 % of cases)[5] in German passives with WERDEN. Secondly, Bredel and Maaß (2016: 313–314) attribute the abovementioned difficulty to morphological factors, given that canonical passive forms (at least in German, English, as well as

4 In this volume, Maaß does not refer only to passives *stricto sensu*, but also to passive-related structures (such as modal infinitives, as may be inferred from an example she provides).

5 Similar estimations are provided by Brinker (1971: 40) and Schoenthal (1976: 124) based on corpus analyses: the former calculated a percentage of 86.32 %, the latter of 84 %. Furthermore, for alternatives to conventional passives agent omission is even more frequent (Lenz 2006: 50). For the English language, estimations were made by Svartvik (1966: 141) and Givón (1979: 58). The former calculated a percentage of 80 % agentless passives, while according to the latter this value reaches 82 % of overall passive forms.

many other languages) are characterised by an analytic structure. In German, particularly, the meaning-carrying part of the verb shifts to the end of the sentence[6]. Similarly, Cutts (2013: 68) states that introducing verbs towards the end of a sentence, as often occurs with passive forms, "forces readers to store large chunks of text in their short-term memory while they wait to discover the doer and what the action will be". Finally, another explanation for this complexity may be the dichotomy "centrality-peripherality" elaborated by Maaß (2015: 78), who recommends using more frequent – and therefore comprehensible – linguistic resources in simplified texts. Although in the quoted paragraph she discusses only more or less common synonyms as well as grammatical categories like genitive, subjunctive, and preterite, the same principle may be applied to passive forms, since, as already mentioned, they are far less frequent than their active counterparts.

Due to the above-discussed reasons, passive forms are generally not recommended in simplified language variants (Easy and Plain Language). For Easy Language, the *Netzwerk Leichte Sprache* (BMAS 2014: 29) as well as Bredel and Maaß (2016: 313–317) recommend against using the passive diathesis. As far as Easy Language Plus (a slightly less simplified language variant) is concerned, Maaß (2020: 244–245) states that passive forms can be used under certain conditions. The variant of Plain Language is less normed than Easy Language; however, some guidelines or recommendations can be found, such as those by Cutts (2013). This author maintains that passive forms are "fostered by bad teaching in schools and universities that equates good writing with formality, obscurity, and Olympian detachment", and even uses disapproving expressions such as "passive-infested style" (ibid.: 63). However, he then moves on to state that the passive voice is still valuable in some cases, since it may serve as a hedging or face-saving strategy, it enables the omission of obvious or irrelevant agents, and thematises important information. Other recommendations for Plain Language (2017) are those written with respect to the text genre pertaining to the medical-pharmaceutical field which will be analysed

6 Also according to Lenz (2006: 74) typical German passive forms are cumbersome due to the verbal bracketing they imply.

here, i.e. layperson summaries of clinical trials; there, it is suggested to avoid the passive diathesis.

In light of these premises, with the passive voice playing an undeniably remarkable role in LSPs but running the risk of affecting comprehensibility, the purpose of this paper is to analyse the aforementioned comprehensibility-enhanced genre in order to point out the frequency of passive forms *lato sensu* as well as their use – and ascertain whether the recommendations are actually followed.

2 Materials and method

The examined comprehensibility-enhanced text genre, i.e. layperson summaries of clinical trials, consists of versions of trial results for non-experts aimed at guaranteeing transparency. These documents, published by pharmaceutical companies in compliance with EU regulation 536/2014, should also be provided with translations in the various languages of the countries that took part in the trial. Clinical trial information for medical experts, by contrast, is only provided in English due to its status of *lingua franca* in science. The present empirical study examines a corpus of English layperson summaries, their German translations, as well as their source texts for experts (trial summaries downloaded directly from the pharmaceutical company websites or, in case these were not published, the analogous information available on the portal ClinicalTrials.gov).

2.1 Automated analysis

The analysis was performed on thirty triplets of texts as indicated above, thus, in total, on ninety texts. The pharmaceutical companies which have produced them are Grünenthal, GSK, Novartis, Bayer, and Boehringer Ingelheim. The rationale for corpus construction was to select texts homogeneously, both in terms of pharmaceutical company and of topic (i.e. pathology to be treated), in order to guarantee that the formulations would be as varied as possible. In this part of the analysis the aim was to pinpoint the frequency of passive sentences.

For this purpose, the software Analyze My Writing[7] and Ratte[8] (Regensburger Analysetool für Texte) were employed as a starting point. As a matter of fact, as will be explained more extensively in 3, these tools sometimes provide both false positives and false negatives. Moreover, Analyze My Writing only signals cases of passives consisting of BE + PAST PARTICIPLE, while Ratte solely marks those with WERDEN + PAST PARTICIPLE. Clearly, this is a great limit of the tools in question, as, especially for German, these are far from all passive forms. The second part of the article therefore aimed at integrating the automated analysis. Another limit is that images, graphs, and tables that could not be copied were not considered.

2.2 Manual analysis

As already mentioned, the aim of this chapter was to complete the automated analysis by considering passive forms that were not identified by the tools Analyze My Writing and Ratte. In German, these include first of all *Zustandspassiv* (or *sein*-passive) as well as the non-canonical *bekommen*-passive[9] (or recipient passive, also with its variants entailing the verbs ERHALTEN and KRIEGEN); in English, passives with the non-canonical auxiliary GET[10] (or similar verbs like BECOME).

Moreover, I decided to analyse other passive-related structures[11], too. Most are specific to German, although some may occur also – or solely – in the Eng-

7 https://www.analyzemywriting.com/

8 https://www.uni-regensburg.de/sprache-literatur-kultur/germanistik-did/downloads/ratte/index.html

9 Zifonun (1992: 254; 1997: 1824) refers to it as "peripheral passive" as opposed to the "central passive" made up by the periphrastic forms with the auxiliaries WERDEN and SEIN, as it does not fulfil all passivity requirements.

10 Cf. e.g. Huddleston/Pullum (2002: 1440–1443); it should be noted that the term "auxiliary" was used exclusively for the sake of simplicity, as its status is debated (cf. *inter alia* Haegeman 1985; Wanner 2013; Puckica 2009).

11 Linguistic literature is replete with terms referring to these phenomena, especially for German. They may be translated as "passive reformulations" (Kolb 1966: 178), "competing forms of passive" or "passive paraphrases" (Helbig/Buscha 1998: 183), "passive variants" (Brinker 1971: 117), "passive synonyms" (Gang 1997), "passive alternatives", "substitute forms of passive" (Puato 2017: 170), and "almost passive constructions" (Weinrich 2005: 163–166). Zifonun (1992; 1997) uses the term "converses" as a hypernym encompassing both standard passives and all other passive-like constructions.

lish language (cf. among others Teich [2012: 213], who underlines that there are fewer passive alternatives in English than in German). The former category encompasses periphrastic structures such as:

- SICH LASSEN + INFINITIVE ("*lassen*-middle" according to e.g. König and Gast [2009: 134–136] and Steinbach [1998: 14]);
- reflexive constructions (called "plain middles" by König and Gast [2009: 134–136] or "middle constructions" by Steinbach [1998]);
- modal infinitives with SEIN[12] (or "tough-movement constructions" according to Steinbach [ibid.: 155], and "modal passives" according to Weinrich [2005: 163–164]);
- GEHÖREN + PAST PARTICIPLE;
- gerundive constructions (also called "modal participles" by Weinrich [2005: 165–166; 542–543]);
- *Funktionsverbgefüge* (empty verb constructions);
- impersonal sentences with the pronoun MAN.

In English, the passive-related forms HAVE + OBJECT + PAST PARTICIPLE and the V-ING passive construction (cf. Puckica 2009 for both) will be considered. Other, more general (non-language-specific) paraphrases include adjectives with a passive connotation and participial attributes.

In chapter 4.2, further considerations about passives will be made with respect to agentivity, their functions and translation.

3 Automated analysis results

The total number of tokens of the analysed corpus was 174,002, with the English and German layperson summaries' subcorpora having 42,309 and 42,108 tokens, respectively, and the trial summaries' subcorpus consisting of 89,585

12 As opposed to the ones with the auxiliary HABEN, which have an active rather than a passive connotation. Some scholars also consider verbs such as STEHEN, BLEIBEN, and GEHEN as variants of SEIN.

tokens. Compared to other corpora which consist of millions of tokens, this corpus is rather small; however, since it consists of texts pertaining to a highly specialised (not concerning general language), quite standardised genre, its size already allows detection of some interesting trends.

The number of passive sentences calculated by the software was always cross-checked manually, as both false positives and false negatives were found. For instance, Analyze My Writing signals constructions with the verb BE + potential PAST PARTICIPLE as passive forms; some incorrectly detected passive phrases contained ADJECTIVES, as in "being constipated", or ADJECTIVES + NOUN PHRASES, as in "There was no excess unmineralized osteoid", "is an unwanted sign", "are known adverse drug reactions", "is a validated instrument". With respect to false negatives, on the other hand, passive forms with the past participle "found" were often overlooked and had to be added manually[13].

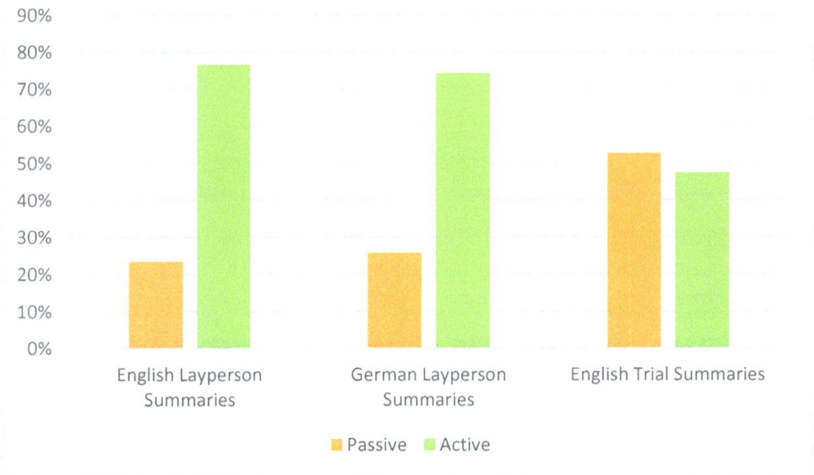

Figure 1: Mean percentages of active and passive sentences

13 With respect to German, it was harder to pinpoint which results were false positives and false negatives, since the software Ratte only calculates the number of passive sentences without listing them explicitly. However, the final values were always corrected, as well, and it may be hypothesised that false positives were made up by the verb WERDEN + ADJECTIVE.

Figure 1 shows the average values of passive and active sentences in the whole corpus. In brief, the trial summaries have an average percentage of passive sentences more than twice as high as the layperson summaries. This trend confirms the initial hypothesis that the passive diathesis would be less frequent in the simplified texts (although it is quite common in absolute terms). The level of passive diathesis is only higher in two layperson summaries than in the respective trial summary. However, the difference is not particularly high: in the first instance, the trial summary passive percentage amounts to 25 %, while that of the English and German layperson summaries amounts to 34.33 % and 36.92 %, respectively. In the second instance, only the German layperson summary has a passive percentage higher than the corresponding trial summary, that is 31.88 % against 28.31 %, while the English layperson summary has a passive percentage of 25 %.

An interesting trend shown both by these instances and Figure 1 is the higher proportion of passive sentences in the German texts than in the English source texts. Overall, 21 out of 30 German texts had more passive sentences than the corresponding English version. This is particularly significant considering that – for this part of the analysis – only the instances of *Vorgangspassiv* were counted in German. If the cases of *Zustandspassiv* had been considered, as well, the discrepancy between the German and English texts would have been even higher, since the semantic difference between statal and processual passives is not marked morphologically in the English language – both are rendered through the verb BE and therefore counted by the software used in the present analysis. Furthermore, initially the level of passive diathesis was expected to decrease, due to the Translation Universal of Simplification (cf. e.g. Baker 1993; Mauranen/Kujamäki 2004). However, some researchers already found that there is a tendency to passivise active constructions in translation (cf. e.g. Bisiada [2019], who analysed English business articles and their German versions).

4 Manual analysis results

As already mentioned in chapter 2.2, this chapter aims at analysing both the features related to passivity which were not considered by the two tools of linguistic analysis, and other aspects deemed to be of interest, such as agentivity and translation of passive structures. With respect to the latter, the purpose was to pinpoint the causes of passive increase in the German texts.

4.1 Missed features in the automated analysis

The first subsection of this chapter examines non-canonical passive constructions as well as alternatives to passives. For the former, the most important phenomenon was found to be *Zustandspassiv*; for the latter, the predominant features occurring in both German and English were attributes (either prenominal or postnominal depending on the language) and adjectives with a passive component. With respect to the German language only, another primary feature was the presence of *Funktionsverbgefüge*.

4.1.1 Passives

As expected, cases of *Zustandspassiv* were extremely frequent (90 occurrences), in particular in metadiscourse and intertextual references, as in "In diesem Abschnitt **sind** die unerwünschten Ereignisse **zusammengefasst**", or "Links zu den Zusammenfassungen **sind** am Ende dieses Dokuments **aufgeführt**". It also occurred in other contexts, as is the case in "Die Aufnahme **war abgeschlossen**" or "Unerwünschte Effekte sind gesundheitliche Beschwerden, die nach Meinung der Ärzte durch [...] **verursacht sind**". A peculiarity of this type of passive, evident in these instances, too, is the absence of an expressed agent, which would be ungrammatical.

The recipient passive (or dative, beneficiary, and addressee passive, cf. Puato 2017: 170–171) was absent in my corpus, both with the verb BEKOMMEN and its variants ERHALTEN and KRIEGEN. This is not particularly surprising considering the constraints of this construction, which may be used if the active sentence from which it stems has both an accusative and a dative object (or a free dative, which may be a *dativus commodi*, a pertinence dative, or even a *dativus incommodi*, cf. ibid.). Even more importantly, this passive form is also subject to diamesic, diaphasic, and diatopic restrictions, since it is generally regarded as a feature of spoken German (Leirbukt 1997) and, depending on the verb choice, it is perceived to be more or less regional and colloquial (Puato 2017: 170–171). The variant with KRIEGEN belongs to a particularly low register, while that with ERHALTEN is stylistically more elevated (ibid.). Further evidence of the relative marginal importance of the recipient passive in LSPs is provided by the fact that, in her meticulous examination of passive forms and passive alternatives in the juridical field, Lenz (2006) did not devote an analysis section to it.

Turning to the English alternatives to the *be*-passive, only one occurrence of the *get*-passive was detected: "When cartilage **gets damaged**, GAG and collagen are also damaged". This low frequency did not come as a surprise, since *get*-passives are by no means as common as *be*-passives: they are perceived to be quite informal and are therefore more frequent in spoken language (cf. *inter alia* Wanner 2013: 47; Puckica 2009: 222; König/Gast 2009: 125). Furthermore, they have semantic constraints: among others, these constructions often allow an adversative reading[14] (König/Gast 2009: 126) – which also characterises the instance provided above – and imply a partial responsibility of the patient (ibid.: 125; Givón/Yang 1994: 119–121). Another verb commutable with BE (cf. Jespersen 1933: 120; Puckica 2009: 222–223) is BECOME, although its status is far more debated than that of GET (ibid.) and it is rarely considered in grammars; in my corpus, only one occurrence was found: "In people with CRVO, the main blood vessel that carries blood away from the retina **becomes blocked**".

4.1.2 Passive alternatives

Starting from passive alternatives specific to the German language, *lassen*-middles did not occur in my corpus. This was to some extent surprising, as it is a rather frequent feature in German (Kunze 1996: 648), especially in the language of science (Puato 2017: 173). With respect to plain middles, on the other hand,

14 Wanner (2013) revisited this claim. In her corpus, two thirds of *get*-passives actually allowed an adversative reading, but she purports that this high percentage was due to the register in which these forms were used.

seven occurrences with the verb "finden" were detected, as in "Weitere Informationen über die Studienergebnisse **finden sich** in den Zusammenfassungen der wissenschaftlichen Ergebnisse".

Modal infinitives with the auxiliary SEIN were not rare (18 occurrences). Most cases entailed the verb phrase "zurückführen auf" and referred to drug effects (or adverse reactions), as in "In dieser Zusammenfassung bezieht sich der Begriff 'Nebenwirkungen' auf diejenigen Ereignisse, die nach Meinung des Studienarztes **auf** das Prüfpräparat **zurückzuführen sein könnten**". Other examples were the following: "Knorpel bestehen aus einer Schicht aus festem, geschmeidigem Gewebe, das in den Zwischenräumen bestimmter Gelenke im Körper, beispielsweise dem Kniegelenk, **vorzufinden ist**", "Manche Arten von Non-Hodgkin-Lymphomen **können** schwer **zu behandeln sein**", and "Asthma gilt als schwer, wenn die Symptome auch dann schwierig **zu kontrollieren sind**, wenn die Patienten Asthma-Medikamente anwenden". Modal infinitives with the verbs STEHEN, BLEIBEN or GEHEN[15] were not found.

A modal connotation, which characterises *lassen*-middles, most plain middles, and (as the name suggests) modal infinitives, is inherent also in the construction GEHÖREN + PAST PARTICIPLE. However, no occurrences were found in my corpus. According to Pape-Müller (1980), this construction is colloquial, which certainly explains its absence. Also, gerundive constructions (or modal participles) have a clear modal component, but they were absent in my corpus as well.

Another passive alternative found in my corpus consists in a subclass of the so-called *Funktionsverbgefüge* (empty verb constructions), contemplated by several grammars and scholars, e.g. by Duden (2016: 562), Weinrich (2005: 164–165), Lenz (2006: 117–152; 247–272), and Puato (2017: 172). The most thorough examination is that by Lenz (2006). Therefore, her model was followed in the present analysis. For verbs such as KOMMEN, GERATEN, and GELANGEN, only active constructions were detected according to her classification, as in "zu den Effekten kommen", "zu Ergebnissen kommen", "zu Ergebnissen gelangen" (18 occurrences altogether). For the verb STEHEN, instead, the pas-

15 The absence of the latter, in particular, does not surprise, as it belongs to a low register (Puato 2017: 172; Vogel 2009).

sive constructions "in Zusammenhang stehen", "in Verbindung stehen", and "zur Verfügung stehen" were quite frequent (35 occurrences), see for instance "Unerwünschte Ereignisse können möglicherweise **in Verbindung** mit den Behandlungen in einer klinischen Prüfung **stehen**". Other instances entail the verbs ERLEBEN (1 occurrence) and BEDÜRFEN (11 occurrences), as in "Ereignisse erleben", "Es bedarf viel Forschung, um herauszufinden, ob [...]". In sum, these cases were quite limited, but this may be related to the general tendency towards verbalisation in comprehensibility-enhanced texts as well as to the fact that the majority of nominalised constructions were active.

To conclude the section devoted solely to German passive alternatives, impersonal constructions with the pronoun MAN were relatively frequent (21 occurrences), too. Some instances from the corpus under analysis are the following: "Weder die Patienten noch die Studienärzte wussten, wer welche Behandlung erhielt. Dies **nennt man** eine doppelt verblindete Studie" or "**Man konnte** jedoch nicht feststellen, ob sich das Medikament stärker auf den Kollagen- oder GAG-Gehalt auswirkte als Placebo". Albeit not meeting all passivity requirements (they may even be passivised, cf. Puato 2017: 171; Helbig 1997), these constructions are agent-averted[16].

As far as English is concerned, four instances of the construction HAVE + OBJECT + PAST PARTICIPLE were detected in the corpus under analysis: "The participants **had their vision checked** every 4 weeks", and "**had pictures of their knee taken** using MRI", just to mention a few. No cases of the V-ING passive construction (or "concealed passive", as in "The house needs painting", cf. Huddleston/Pullum [2002: 1199–1200]) were found. Indeed, besides having aspectual differences with the canonical passive, this form is far less frequent (Puckica 2009: 226).

Turning to cross-linguistic passive alternatives, adjectives with a passive component – which have a modal connotation, as well (cf. Puato 2017: 173) – were found in both examined languages. In German, the suffixes *-lich* and *-bar* were quite productive. With respect to the former (24 occurrences), instances like "zugänglich", "erhältlich", "verträglich", and "verständlich" were found. As

16 Unlike for many other passives and passive alternatives, here agent expression is not only superfluous, but even ungrammatical.

far as the -*bar* suffix (19 occurrences) is concerned, some examples are "tolerierbar", "verfügbar", "vorstellbar", "unschätzbar", "vorhersehbar", "erkennbar", and "vergleichbar". Other passive pseudosuffixes listed by Lenz (2006: 169–186) and Puato (2017: 173) are -*wert*, -*würdig*, -*fertig*, -*bereit*, -*bedürftig*, -*pflichtig*, -*fähig*. However, none of these were found, except for -*fertig* ("gebrauchsfertig", 2 occurrences) and -*fähig*, but the latter occurred only in an active adjective, i.e. "gebärfähig" (1 occurrence). This distribution approximately corresponds to that detected by Lenz (2006: 170), who noted that the most frequent adjectives are those with the suffixes -*bar* and -*lich*, followed by -*wert*, -*pflichtig*, -*bedürftig*, and -*würdig*. Finally, another suffix detected in the present corpus is -*abel*, as in "resektabel", a technical term found in an intertextual reference from one layperson summary to its corresponding trial summary and its original title. In English, suffixes making up passive adjectives are -*able*, -*ible*, and -*uble* (e.g. Haspelmath 1994: 163; Puckica 2009: 229–233). Of these, only the former occurred in my corpus, i.e. in the adjectives "available" or "applicable" (44 occurrences altogether). This distribution is not particularly surprising, in that -*able* is nowadays the only productive suffix out of this group (ibid.: 230).

As far as participial attributes expressing passivity are concerned, so-called *Linksattribute*, that is prenominal attributes, were frequent in German (137 occurrences). Some of these built quite complex nominal phrases, as in "Nebenwirkungen des **auf den chirurgischen Schnitten und Wunden verwendeten** Klebers", "Angabe der **mit den vorstehend genannten Hyperlinks verknüpften** Websites", "die **von Ihnen angewendeten medizinischen** Behandlungen". In English, such prenominal attributes occurred more seldomly, in only 44 cases (e.g. "total **planned** dose", "other **commonly used** methods", "**approved** type"); postnominal attributes (or "bare passives" according to Huddleston/Pullum [2002: 1429–1430]), such as "adverse events **caused by the trial drugs**", or "condition **brought on by a sudden decrease in blood flow to the heart muscles**", were far more frequent (228 occurrences). Indeed, these may be considered the English equivalent of German *Linksattribute*, as English prenominal attributes – unlike postmodifiers – cannot be expanded to reach a certain degree of complexity (cf. Fabricius-Hansen 2010: 5). Participial phrases (separated by a comma, signalling their non-restrictiveness) were found relatively often, too (36 occurrences), as in "gastrointestinal stromal tumors, **ab-**

breviated with GIST" or "autologous chondrocyte implantation, **also known as ACI surgery**"; some instances occurred in German, as well, albeit not as frequently (17 occurrences). As a matter of fact, these constructions constitute a common alternative to relative clauses only in English (ibid.: 7). All of them undoubtedly contribute to text concision.

4.2 Further considerations: agents, functions, translation

What was stated in chapter 1.3 with respect to agent omission was confirmed in my corpus, as well. The overwhelming majority of analysed passives did not have overt agents[17]. This concerns cases where the agent was obvious and inferable on the basis of encyclopaedic knowledge, as in "[...] gastrointestinal stromal tumors, abbreviated with GIST, that had spread to other parts of the body or could not be removed" or "The placebo was taken as a tablet by mouth", where the implicit agents are doctors or surgeons and trial participants, respectively. Another reason is the expression of the agent in the same sentence or paragraph, but not as an explicit argument headed by the preposition "by" (or "von" in German), as is the case in "**The doctors** did a CT or MRI scan of the participants' tumors every 4 weeks for the first 3 months, then every 6 weeks for the next 3 months. After that, the tumors were checked every 8 weeks [...]". Finally, another cause of agentlessness is the general nature of the agent itself in some statements, which makes it superfluous, as in "These medical problems are called 'adverse events'". In this instance the agent, if explicit, should have been "doctors" or "all doctors", which would have been slightly pedantic – although in layperson summaries technical terms are often signalled by expressions such as "doctors call these + TERM" after cataphoric definitions.

When the agent was expressed, it was generally highlighted, i.e. its semantic value was to underline that the action was carried out by it and not by other individuals or objects (cf. Scarpa 2008: 46), as in "All serious side effects were

17 For the sake of simplicity and concision, all instances and considerations at the beginning of this chapter are in English, the source language, but they are valid also for German, in that, as we will see in the paragraphs concerning translation, this language did not add any agents, but rather tended to *omit* them when it transformed English active sentences into passive ones.

reported by less than 1 % of patients in either treatment group" or "If the study doctor thinks that an adverse event was caused by the study medicine, they record this as a possible side effect (adverse reaction)". In other – more limited – cases, it was expressed only since it was not omissible (cf. Huddleston/ Pullum 2002: 1428), as occurs in this example involving the verb *follow* with a temporal reading: "This 4-week period was followed by 27 days of no doses".

Overall, the functions of passives were mainly to focus on patients rather than agents, in case these were too obvious or not important, as seen above, or to avoid the repetitive use of excessively similar constructions. Another cause is theme-rheme progression. With respect to the second instance provided in the previous paragraph, for example, *adverse events* makes up the theme, discussed in depth in the previous pages ("Given"), while *the study medicine* is the rheme ("New"). This progression is enabled by the use of a passive form. Furthermore, another stylistic cause consists in the concision allowed by passives, which are frequently found in titles and tables, where there is often no room for wordiness.

As mentioned above and in 1.3, passives are tightly intertwined with depersonalisation and anonymisation, which are often of utmost importance in medicine – and science in general. Frequent exceptions to this principle were detected in my corpus: see, for instance "The researchers randomly assigned the participants [...]", or even "We did statistical tests on these results" and "We also measured the time from starting the study treatment until the patients died".

Another interesting feature that I decided to look at was the increase in passives in German highlighted by the automated analysis. Firstly, it was found that the higher number of passives in this language was often due to recourse to relative clauses containing a passive verb to translate English postmodifiers[18], which, as already stated in 4.1.2, are ungrammatical in German. See, for instance, the following translations: "Proteine [...], die als Autoantikörper

18 Another frequent way of translating such postmodifiers, mentioned in 4.1.2, consists in *Linksattribute*, their German equivalent. See, for instance, the German translation "mit einer **als Schuppen bezeichneten** silbrig-weißen Anhäufung bedeckt" from "covered with silvery white buildup **called scales**".

bezeichnet werden" (from the source text "Proteins called autoantibodies") or "die Patienten, die in diese Studie aufgenommen wurden" (from "patients included in this study"). In another excerpt, a postmodifier was translated similarly, although not with a relative clause: "In dieser Studie wurden zwei Medikamente verabreicht" from the source text "The drugs given in this trial were […]". Clearly, these English instances had a passive component, too, but – unlike their German translation – they were not subsumable under the category of canonical passives.

In other cases, though, passivity was lacking completely in the source text and was added in the target one. Some instances of this phenomenon, which will be called "passives *ex nihilo*", were the following: "Medikamente, mit denen Schmerzen und Entzündungen behandelt werden können" from "medicines that can lower pain and inflammation", "Im Rahmen dieser Studie sollten neue Erkenntnisse über die Wirkung und Sicherheit von […] gewonnen werden" from "The purpose of this trial was to learn about the effects and safety of […]". Here, in addition to the passive transformation, a difficulty is posed by the use of an empty verb construction rather than an easier verb such as "erfahren". In many cases, passives *ex nihilo* went hand in hand with agent omission, as in "Bei diesem Termin wurden Blut- und Urinproben entnommen" from "Trial staff took blood and urine samples at some of the trial visits" or "Es wird nach einer besseren Möglichkeit zur Behandlung von Patienten […] gesucht" from "Researchers are looking for a better way to treat […]". Agents were kept only if strictly necessary, as in "Das zugewiesene Medikament wurde von den Teilnehmern […] selbst unter die Haut gespritzt" from "Participants took their assigned treatment by giving themselves an injection under the skin". However, I suggest that this strategy be avoided. As a matter of fact, beside affecting comprehensibility, it also impacts on the interpersonal function of language, since in the source text the mention of the agent (be it *researchers*, *trial staff* etc.) also helps build trust and increase authoritativeness.

Finally, some instances of passives *ex nihilo* were due to structural differences between English and German rather than translators' personal – arbitrary – choices, as in "test positive" and "positiv getestet werden".

5 Conclusions

In sum, the number of passive sentences was lower in the comprehensibility-enhanced texts for non-experts than in the trial summaries, but it was still quite high, despite the recommendations existing in the field. Most of them did not contain overt agents, which conflicts with the action orientation and agent explicitation recommended by Maaß (2015: 78–80); at the same time, though, they were mostly still easily inferable and did not lead to significant interpretation issues. Furthermore, canonical constructions were undoubtedly more frequent than non-prototypical ones or passive alternatives. This distribution may be explained through the dichotomy "centrality-peripherality" by Maaß (ibid.), already mentioned in 1.3, according to which more frequent linguistic resources should be favoured over sporadically occurring ones. A second reason, specific to German translated texts, is interference, that is a certain tendency to repeat constructions found in the source text rather than replacing them with more natural-sounding, idiomatic ones in the target language. As we have seen in 2.2 and 4.1, non-prototypical passives and, even more so, passive alternatives are much sparser in English than in German. Therefore, the majority of passives in the source language are ascribable to canonical passives, and this distribution may have contributed to the high number of prototypical passives in the target language, as well. Clearly, there are plenty of exceptions to this statement, since even in translation, constructions specific solely to the target language may be found (cf. e.g. Kunze [1996: 684–688] and the use of *lassen* middles in German translations from English). In my corpus, too, some peripheral constructions did occur, but without exceeding expectations and respecting all diamesic and diaphasic constraints. In conclusion, a further research desideratum could be to examine users' reception and elaboration of passive constructions and alternatives to passive in these texts.

Literature

Alexiadou, Artemis/Schäfer, Florian (eds.) (2013): *Non-Canonical Passives.* Amsterdam/Philadelphia: John Benjamins.

Baker, Mona (1993): "Corpus linguistics and translation studies – Implications and applications". In: Baker, Mona/Francis, Gill/Tognini-Bonelli, Elena (eds.): *Text and Technology. In Honour of John Sinclair.* Amsterdam: John Benjamins, pp. 233–250.

Bisiada, Mario (2019): "Translated language or edited language? A study of passive constructions in translation manuscripts and their published versions". In: *Across Languages and Cultures* 20: 1, pp. 35–56.

BMAS (2014): "Leichte Sprache. Ein Ratgeber". In: https://www.bmas.de/DE/Service/Publikationen/a752-leichte-sprache-ratgeber.html (last accessed 23 June 2021).

Bredel, Ursula/Maaß, Christiane (2016): *Leichte Sprache. Theoretische Grundlagen, Orientierung für die Praxis.* Berlin: Dudenverlag.

Brinker, Klaus (1971): *Das Passiv im heutigen Deutsch. Form und Funktion.* München: Max Hueber Verlag.

Chomsky, Noam (1957): *Syntactic Structures.* The Hague/Paris: Mouton.

Cooreman, Ann (1994): "A functional typology of antipassives". In: Fox, Barbara/Hopper, Paul J. (eds.): *Voice. Form and Function.* Amsterdam: John Benjamins, pp. 49–88.

Cutts, Martin (2013): *Oxford Guide to Plain English.* 4th ed. Oxford: Oxford University Press.

Duden (2016): *Duden. Die Grammatik.* 9th ed. Vol. 4. Berlin: Dudenverlag.

European Medicines Agency (2017): "Recommendations of the expert group on clinical trials for the implementation of Regulation (EU) No 536/2014 on clinical trials on medicinal products for human use, Version 2". In: https://ec.europa.eu/health/sites/default/files/files/eudralex/vol-10/2017_01_26_summaries_of_ct_results_for_laypersons.pdf (last accessed 22 August 2021).

Fabricius-Hansen, Cathrine (2010): "Adjektiv-/Partizipialattribute im diskursbezogenen Kontrast (Deutsch – Englisch/Norwegisch)". In: *Deutsche Sprache* 38, pp. 175–192.

Gang, Gook-Jin (1997): *Passivsynonyme als Elemente der wissenschaftlichen Fachsprache im Deutschen.* Frankfurt am Main: Peter Lang.

Givón, Talmy (1979): *On Understanding Grammar*. New York: Academic Press.

Givón, Talmy/Yang, Lynne (1994): "The rise of the English GET-passive". In: Fox, Barbara/Hopper, Paul J. (eds.): *Voice: Form and Function*. Amsterdam/Philadelphia: John Benjamins, pp. 119–150.

Grimm, Hannelore (1975): "Verstehen, Imitation und Produktion von Passivsätzen". In: Grimm, Hannelore/Schöler, Hermann/Wintermantel, Margret (eds.): *Zur Entwicklung sprachlicher Strukturformen bei Kindern*. Weinheim: Beltz, pp. 73–99.

Haegeman, Liliane (1985): "The get-passive and burzio's generalization". In: *Lingua* 66: 1, pp. 53–77.

Halliday, Michael A. K. (1990): "The construction of knowledge and value in the grammar of scientific discourse: With reference to Charles Darwin's 'The origin of species'". In: De Stasio, Clotilde/Gotti, Maurizio/Bonadei, Rossana (eds.): *La rappresentazione verbale e iconica: valori estetici e funzionali*. Milano: Guerini, pp. 57–80.

Haspelmath, Martin (1994): "Passive participles across languages". In: Fox, Barbara/Hopper, Paul J. (eds.): *Voice: Form and Function*. Amsterdam/Philadelphia: John Benjamins, pp. 151–178.

Helbig, Gerhard (1997): "'Man'-Konstruktionen und/oder Passiv?" In: *Deutsch als Fremdsprache* 26, pp. 82–85.

Helbig, Gerhard/Buscha, Joachim (1998): *Deutsche Grammatik. Ein Handbuch für den Ausländerunterricht*. Leipzig: Langenscheidt.

Huddleston, Rodney/Pullum, Geoffrey K. (2002): *The Cambridge Grammar of the English Language*. Cambridge: Cambridge University Press.

Jespersen, Otto (1933): *Essentials of English Grammar*. London: G. Allen and Unwin Ltd.

Kolb, Herbert (1966): "Das verkleidete Passiv. Über Passivumschreibungen im modernen Deutsch". In: *Sprache im technischen Zeitalter* 19, pp. 173–198.

König, Ekkehard/Gast, Volker (2009): *Understanding English-German Contrasts*. Berlin: Erich Schmidt Verlag.

Kunze, Jürgen (1996): "Plain middles and *lassen* middles in German: reflexive constructions and sentence perspective". In: *Linguistics* 34, pp. 645–695.

Leirbukt, Oddleif (1997): *Untersuchungen zum 'bekommen'-Passiv im heutigen Deutsch*. Tübingen: Niemeyer.

Leiss, Elisabeth (1992): *Die Verbalkategorien des Deutschen. Ein Beitrag zur Theorie der sprachlichen Kategorisierung*. Berlin/New York: Walter de Gruyter.

Lenz, Magdalena (2006): *Grammatik und Stil: Das Passiv als stilistisches Mittel im Vergleich zu konkurrierenden grammatischen Konstruktionen*. Unpublished PhD dissertation, Technische Universität Berlin, Fakultät I-Geisteswissenschaften.

Maaß, Christiane (2015): *Leichte Sprache. Das Regelbuch*. Münster: Lit-Verlag.

Maaß, Christiane (2020): *Easy Language – Plain Language – Easy Language Plus. Balancing Comprehensibility and Acceptability*. Berlin: Frank & Timme.

Magris, Marella (1992): "La traduzione del linguaggio medico: analisi contrastiva di testi in lingua italiana, inglese e tedesca". In: Di Mauro, Gabriella/Scarpa, Federica (eds.): *Traduzione, società e cultura*. Vol. 2, pp. 3–82.

Mauranen, Anna/Kujamäki, Pekka (2004): *Translation Universals. Do They Exist?*. Amsterdam: John Benjamins.

Pape-Müller, Sabine (1980): *Textfunktionen des Passivs. Untersuchungen zur Verwendung von grammatisch-lexikalischen Passivformen*. Tübingen: Niemeyer.

Perlmutter, David M./Postal, Paul M. (1983): "Some proposed laws of basic clause structure". In: Perlmutter, David M. (ed.): *Studies in Relational Grammar 1*. Chicago: University of Chicago Press, pp. 81–128.

Puato, Daniela (2017): "Diathese II: Passivalternativen". In: Puato, Daniela/Di Meola, Claudio (eds.): *DaF-Übungsgrammatiken zwischen Sprachwissenschaft und Didaktik: Perspektiven auf die semanto-pragmatische Dimension der Grammatik*. Frankfurt am Main: Peter Lang, pp. 169–184.

Puckica, Jérôme (2009): "Passive constructions in Present-Day English". In: *Groninger Arbeiten zur Germanistischen Linguistik* 49, pp. 215–235.

Roelcke, Thorsten (1999): *Fachsprachen*. Berlin: Erich Schmidt Verlag.

Sager, Juan C./Dungworth, David/McDonald, Peter F. (1980): *English Special Languages: Principles and Practice in Science and Technology*. Wiesbaden: Oscar Brandstetter Verlag.

Scarpa, Federica (2008): *La traduzione specializzata. Un approccio didattico professionale*. 2nd ed. Milano: Hoepli.

Schoenthal, Gisela (1976): *Das Passiv in der deutschen Standardsprache*. München: Max Hueber Verlag.

Shibatani, Masayoshi (1988): "Introduction". In: Shibatani, Masayoshi (ed.): *Passive and Voice*. Amsterdam/Philadelphia: John Benjamins, pp. 3–8.

Steinbach, Markus (1998): *Middles in German*. Unpublished PhD dissertation, Humboldt-Universität zu Berlin, Philosophische Fakultät II.

Svartvik, Jan (1966): *On Voice in the English Verb*. The Hague/Paris: Mouton & Co.

Teich, Elke (2012): *Cross-Linguistic Variation in System and Text. A Methodology for the Investigation of Translations and Comparable Texts*. Berlin: Walter de Gruyter.

Vogel, Petra M. (2009): "Passiv". In: Hentschel, Elke/Vogel, Petra M. (eds.): *Deutsche Morphologie*. Berlin/New York: Walter de Gruyter, pp. 282–296.

Wanner, Anja (2013): "The *get*-passive at the intersection of *get* and the passive". In: Alexiadou, Artemis/Schäfer, Florian (eds.): *Non-Canonical Passives*. Amsterdam/Philadelphia: John Benjamins, pp. 43–62.

Weinrich, Harald (2005): *Textgrammatik der deutschen Sprache*. 3rd ed. Hildesheim/Zürich/New York: Georg Olms Verlag.

Wunderlich, Dieter (1993): "Diathesen". In: Jacobs, Joachim/von Stechow, Arnim/Sternefeld, Wolfgang/Vennemann, Theo (eds.): *Syntax. Ein internationales Handbuch zeitgenössischer Forschung/An International Handbook of Contemporary Research*. Vol. 1. Berlin/New York: Walter de Gruyter, pp. 730–747.

Zifonun, Gisela (1992): "Das Passiv im Deutschen: Agenten, Blockaden und (De-) Gradierungen". In: Hoffmann, Ludger (ed.): *Deutsche Syntax: Ansichten und Aussichten*. Berlin/New York: Walter de Gruyter, pp. 250–275.

Zifonun, Gisela (1997): "Das Passiv (und die Familie der grammatischen Konversen)". In: Zifonun, Gisela/Hoffmann, Ludger/Strecker, Bruno (eds.): *Grammatik der deutschen Sprache*. Berlin/New York: Walter de Gruyter, pp. 1789–1858.

Isabel Rink / Rebecca Schulz

Data collection in the field of Accessible Health Communication

1 Introduction

As a reaction to the results of the health literacy study conducted by Schaeffer et al. (2018) in Germany, which show that more than half of the German population state that they have problems in finding, understanding and applying health information, the National Action Plan Health Literacy was released. It is a catalogue of 15 suggestions that aim at improving health literacy within the German population. With regard to this article, suggestions 8 and 9 of the catalogue are exceedingly relevant: *8) Improving* ***communication*** *between health professionals and users in a comprehensible and effective manner.* This improvement of communication becomes more concrete in suggestion *9)* where it is proposed to *make health information more user-friendly* which can be achieved by reducing complexity through the use of Plain Language (Schaeffer et al. 2018: 41–42; own translation).

Plain Language can be defined as a variety of German located in the field of accessible communication that serves to overcome communication barriers (Maaß 2020; for an overview see Maaß/Rink 2019). Communication barriers may affect the accessibility of information whether it is oral or written, online or offline. In contrast to standard or even expert language, Plain Language is a strategically reduced form of German leading to more accessibility, more perceptibility, more comprehensibility and more acceptability and can therefore be processed more easily by non-experts (Maaß 2020: 13). Especially non-experts with diverse communicative needs, e.g. people with cognitive impairments, who are often part of vulnerable groups (Schaeffer et al. 2018: 39; also see chapter 2.1) may benefit by this adapted language variety (Rink 2020: 107ff.; 178ff.). Thus, Plain Language is supposed to improve access to health information that, in the field of health communication, is regulated by law, inter alia, in the Convention on the Rights of Persons with Disabilities (2006). Pursuant to article 25:

> States Parties shall take all appropriate measures to ensure access for persons with disabilities to health services that are gender-sensitive, including health-related rehabilitation.

In particular, this includes:

- the same range, quality and standard of free or affordable health care and programmes as provided to other persons
- providing the health services needed by persons with disabilities specifically because of their disabilities
- providing the health services as close as possible to people's own communities
- requiring health professionals to provide care of the same quality to persons with disabilities
- prohibiting discrimination against persons with disabilities in the provision of health and life insurance
- preventing discriminatory denial of health care or health services or food and fluids on the basis of disability. (CRPD 2006: 18)

Accessible health communication as a subfield of accessible communication is still lacking valid results from research with vulnerable groups and especially from research with people with cognitive impairments. This will be in the focus in the following chapter.

2 Conducting research with people with cognitive impairments and data collection methods

One output of research on accessible communication in recent years has been that empirical data on people with disabilities and especially on people with cognitive impairments are still very undifferentiated. One desideratum is research on the health situation and literacy of people with cognitive impairments, also because participation in health issues is a human right (see Chapter 1 and CRPD Article 25). The focus of this chapter is on people with cognitive impairments who – among the people with disabilities – have a special need for accessible health information and communication (see also Maaß/Rink 2022).

While research on the health literacy of the German population shows requirements regarding the needs for health information and communication, findings on the health literacy of people with cognitive impairments are still lacking. One step towards closing this gap is the study conducted by Schulz (in preparation) on understanding and retaining health information. With recourse to previous studies (see for example Gutermuth 2020, Rathmann/Dadaczynski 2020, Rathmann et al. 2021) this article aims at emphasising the necessity for adapting data collection methods, and related to this, the procedure of data collection in research with people with cognitive impairments.

2.1 People with cognitive impairments

Following Fornefeld (2002: 44; own translation) people with cognitive impairments are limited in the analysis and synthesis of perception, experience, recognition and understanding due to brain damage that also affects learning and an active lifestyle as a whole. For the German context, people with cognitive impairments often have a limited reading competence (see Ratz 2013, Bredel/Maaß 2016, Rink 2020). "No more than approximately 30 % of the people with cognitive disabilities are readers in the sense of reading texts" (Maaß 2020: 54; Günthner 1999). Nearly 70 percent of people with cognitive impairments are not able to read properly (i.e. extract meaning) and therefore depend on the help of others in order to access information (Bredel/Maaß 2016: 153). Ratz (2013: 343ff.) conducted a study at Bavarian schools focussing on pupils with limited intellectual development. He came to a similar result showing that almost 33 percent of the pupils (13 years old) are able to read properly (extract meaning) at all, meaning that reading becomes an automatic process in which words and syllables can be recognised at one glance. Reading competence that includes extracting the meaning of information however is necessary for independent participation without the help of third parties. Another study on reading and text comprehension was conducted by Bock/Lange (2017) focussing on adults with cognitive impairments. However, the size of the sampling was not sufficient to gain significance. The above mentioned studies lead to the conclusion that there is a major need for research focussing on people with special communicative needs.

All results show that these people with cognitive impairments who have limited reading skills also show reduced "global, grammatical and discourse knowledge" (Maaß 2020: 92). This reduced common knowledge often also results in poor health literacy that does not only affect people with cognitive impairments but all groups designated as *vulnerable*. These include the following target groups (Schaeffer et al 2018: 39):

- people with low sociocultural and economic resources
- people with migration background
- people with chronic diseases
- people in higher age brackets (65 years and older)

These groups are recognised as having a lower health literacy in comparison to the general population (ibid.) as they are confronted with difficulties when dealing with health related information particularly often (ibid: 97). Furthermore, people with a lower health literacy are more likely to have worse health, but a higher risk for accompanying and secondary diseases (Rathmann et al. 2021: 1). In summary, Geukes (2019: 5) states: Vulnerable groups can only make decisions on health issues according to their ability to understand and process (mostly written) information. This means that health information has to be comprehensible and processable in order to enable people to act, thus to make decisions, in a second step.

Research shows that a cognitive impairment goes hand in hand with an impairment of intelligence (see Häßler/Eggers 2012; Schuppener/Bock 2019; Seidel 2013) which is an important aspect in the field of health communication. In this context, self-assessments of people with an IQ below 80 are not reliable anymore (Zerssen 1975 cited from Lehrl 2018: 9). Furthermore, people with average intelligence have greater medical knowledge than people with a lower

IQ (Schmidt et al. 1979 cited from Lehrl 2018: 9). As was shown, people with cognitive impairments have limited linguistic and cognitive competences due to brain damage. This severely affects their intellectual abilities including the analysis and synthesis of perception, experiences, understanding and recognition. In turn, this has consequences for their learning behaviour and way of life (Fornefeld 2002: 44).

Despite these findings, people with cognitive impairments are only rarely taken into account in research, especially in the field of participative research on health issues. Rathmann et al. (2021: 2) name the lack of appropriate data collection methods as one possible reason for this desideratum. Texts, either online or offline, oral or written, being part of the data collection setting, are used for knowledge capturing and processing. However, texts have certain features that are not yet being taken into account in research with people with special communicative needs. Recent studies show that the research on accessible communication can contribute to the adaptation of data collection methods to the linguistic and cognitive abilities and special communicative needs of people with cognitive impairments.

2.2 Data collection methods and standardisation

Data collection methods are usually standardised to allow comparability between different target groups (Bortz/Döring 2016). In the empirical research on accessible communication there are different methods that are applied depending on the research question and aim of the study. With recourse to previous and recent studies (see Gutermuth 2020, Deilen 2022, Schulz in preparation, Ahrens in preparation, Keller in preparation) with primary target groups of Easy Language and Plain Language, these can be: eyetracking, free recall, rating and questionnaires.

Research on Accessible Communication on both sides, text and user perspectives (see Chapter 1 in this volume), has shown that these methods are not yet adapted to the cognitive and linguistic prerequisites of people with cognitive impairments. These methods were designed by experts with diverging abilities, but lacking the knowledge concerning the communicative needs of people with cognitive impairments as participants. Most of the time, data gathering processes take place in an expert-non-expert-context in which the knowledge of the two persons concerning the subject differs significantly (common ground, see Clark 1996). This is because the expert or, in terms of the data gathering process, the researcher has a different structured knowledge with regard to the subject and thus the language used in this concrete situation than can be expected from non-experts and especially from people with linguistic or cognitive impairments (Bromme/Jucks/Rambow 2004: 114f.; Rink 2020: 175ff.). In order to help close this gap, guidance for the adaptation of data collection methods can be provided by the approach used in intralingual translation where Easy Language and Plain Language are strategically applied in order to enable access to content at eye level for people with special communicative needs. By means of complexity-reduced language, the common ground between the expert and the non-expert or the researcher and the participant or the sender and the addressee is supposed to be increased (see for example Hansen-Schirra/Maaß 2019, Maaß 2020, Rink 2020; also see Chapter 1 in this volume).

The aim is to compensate for a possible asymmetry of knowledge in order to get valid results which means using a language – carrying information, whether oral or written – in a way that meets the cognitive prerequisites and the knowledge of non-experts. Rink (2020: 180f.; Maaß/Rink 2020) identifies linguistic, conceptual and medial strategies which help to overcome barriers in texts – oral or written – and facilitate access to content in order to enable users to act on given information. These strategies will be applied for the adaptation of the data collection methods in chapter 4. The aim of this subchapter was to demonstrate the necessity for adaptation of data gathering methods for people with cognitive impairments. In the following, the focus is on selected data gathering methods and recommendations for research with this group as participants.

2.3 Data collection methods and adaptation with regard to participants with special communicative needs

In many research disciplines, the typical data collection process is located on the user side not taking into consideration the particular linguistic and cognitive abilities and therefore, special communicative needs of people with cognitive impairments as necessary prerequisites for reliable outcomes. By contrast, the *Hildesheim school's accessible communication model* (Maaß/Rink 2019; chapter 1 in this volume) focuses on the text perspective in the first step, meaning that accessible content (as a text characteristic) is a prerequisite for participation on the part of the user. That is only possible if the data collection methods are adapted to the special needs of participants with communicative impairments, respectively cognitive impairments. This means that linguistic, conceptual and medial adaptations are required when effectiveness is the aim of reliable data collection. According to this approach, the different data collection methods have to first be adapted before the investigation to facilitate reliable conclusions.

In the last few months, there was an increase in the number of requests for language optimization received by the German Research Centre for Easy Language (2021). These requests refer to e.g. questionnaires or anamnesis forms. However, language optimization does not always relate to the needs of people with impairments, showing that even participants with average reading skills have difficulties in dealing with standardised data collection methods and/or complex content. Therefore, effectiveness requires appropriate data collection methods, meaning that they have to meet the special cognitive and linguistic needs of non-experts.

3 Methodology and application

Rathmann et al. (2021) state that in their study almost 64 % percent of people with a disability have difficulties in finding, understanding, assessing and applying health information. This is not just an issue for the group mentioned but can be(come) a problem that affects a whole population i.e. when a disease or pandemic leads to conditions where accessible health information, respectively communication, is a necessary part of crisis management. In this case, the population of a whole country and beyond relies on accessible health information as it is claimed in article 25 of the CRPD and NAP, recommendations 8 and 9 (see chapter 2).

However, accessibility includes an adaptation of content to the needs of diverse target groups. One way of adaptation is the Hildesheim school's accessible communication model (see Ahrens et al. in this volume) according to which the text perspective is to be taken into account first in order to examine the user perspective including effectiveness of the information in a second step. As was shown in chapters 2.1 and 2.3, the data collection methods have to be adapted for research with people with disabilities and especially with people with cognitive impairments as their reading abilities are often very limited (see Ratz 2013, Bredel/Maaß 2016, Rink 2020).

In the following chapter, the focus is on concrete methods that were applied in the study by Schulz (in preparation) on how health information is understood and retained by people with cognitive impairments. With regard to health literacy, understanding and retaining are important prerequisites to enable users to act on the basis of the information given. In the next subchapters the respective method is presented, followed by a demonstration of problems with regard to the special needs of this target group and suggestions for the adaptation. These suggestions are based on the linguistic, conceptual and medial strategies according to Rink (2020) (see chapter 2.2).

3.1 Neuropsychological assessment

The study this article relates to is based on six standardised tests that aim at determining the participants' cognitive performance. Depending on the individual test, the emphasis is put on a certain aspect of this cognitive performance, which will be presented in this subchapter. The results of these tests are then correlated with results gained from the other methodological steps in the sense of data triangulation (see Bortz/Döring 2016; Flick 2011). The advantage is the generation of precise data with regard to the specific individual by means of an interrelation of the respective results. Specifically, the test series is composed as follows (shown here in the order in which they were performed):

- Trail Making Test A+B (TMT)
- Repeating Sequences of Numbers
- Regensburg Word Fluency Test (RWT)

- Multiple-Choice Vocabulary Test Part B
- Salzburg Reading Screening
- Verbal Learning and Memory Test

In the following, these tests are briefly presented. Then, as an example, the Regensburg Word Fluency Test is used to show possible difficulties that can arise and which adaptations are necessary for research with people with cognitive impairments.

TMT-A and TMT-B

The Trail Making Test examines the visual-motor-speed, working memory and attention span (Tischler/Petermann 2010: 79). It consists of parts A and B. In part A, the numbers 1 to 25 are arranged on an A4 sheet and are to be connected in ascending order by the participant. In TMT part B, there are not only numbers (1–13), but also letters (A–L) that also have to be connected (1A–2B–3C). The aim is to complete this task as fast as possible.

Repeating Sequences of Numbers

This test is one of eleven subtests from the German adaptation of the Wechsler Adult Intelligence Scale. It aims at examining the capacity of the working memory and consists of two parts (Petermann 2008). In the first part, the participant has to repeat the sequence of numbers in the same way in which it was orally presented by the investigator. The amount of numbers per sequence increases from two numbers to nine. In the second part, the participant has to repeat the numbers in reverse order. The shortest sequence in this part consists of two numbers, the longest one of eight.

Multiple-Choice Vocabulary Test Part B

This test examines the general level of intelligence and consists of 37 rows with 5 words each in which the participant has to recognise and underline the word that actually exists (Lehrl 2018: 13, 17). The complexity of the words increases from the first to the last row (ibid.: 32).

Salzburg Reading Screening

The Salzburg Reading Screening was originally designed for the application in German schools, grades 2 to 9. It examines the basal reading level (Wimmer/Mayringer 2019: 9). Within three minutes, the participant must evaluate as many sentences as possible in terms of correctness by circling a checkmark or cross. Wimmer/Mayringer (ibid.: 17) state that the catalogue of sentences was chosen in such a way that the participants' prerequisites do not cause any problems for the evaluation. This aspect is considered in more detail in Schulz (in preparation).

Verbal Learning and Memory Test

The Verbal Learning and Memory Test examines the performance of the memory. In a total of 5 runs, a learning list of 15 words is read to the participant of which he/she has to recall as many words as possible after each run. After a break of 30 minutes, this recall takes place again in order to see how many words the participant retained. Furthermore, the investigator reads out a second list and the participant has to say whether the word belongs to the learning list or not (Helmstaedter/Lendt/Lux 2001: 16).

Regensburger Wortflüssigkeitstest (RWT) – Regensburg Word Fluency Test

This test was originally used in the diagnosis of patients with acquired brain damage in order to examine divergent thinking. Divergent thinking means fluent, original thinking aimed at producing as many potential solutions as possible (Aschenbrenner/Tucha/Lange 2000: 5). According to specific rules, the participant must name as many words as possible beginning with a certain letter within two minutes (ibid.: 9). The word fluency test consists of four parts examining formal-lexical word fluency (with and without change of category) and semantic word fluency (with and without change of category).

As already mentioned at the beginning of this chapter, the tests of this neuropsychological assessment are standardised. For their execution, there are instructions given in the manuals of each test which the investigator can use as a guide. With regard to research with people with cognitive impairments, the challenge is to explain the task or the rules in an accessible manner. This will be shown in the following, using the Regensburg Word Fluency Test as an example. There, the instruction for the formal lexical word fluency for the letter 'S' is as follows (Aschenbrenner/Tucha/Lange 2000: 15):

- Dabei sollen Sie keine Wörter mehrfach nennen.

  You should not name any words more than once (translation Schulz)

- Die Wörter dürfen aber nicht mit den gleichen Wortstamm beginnen, also 'Sport – Sporthose – Sportplatz – Sportschuhe' gelten nur als ein Wort.

  The words must not start with the same root, so 'sports – sports pants – sports field – sports shoes' count as only one word (translation Schulz)

- Weiterhin dürfen Sie auch keine Eigennamen nennen, also 'Stefan – Susanne – Stuttgart – Schweiz' gelten nicht.

  You are not allowed to use proper names, so 'Stefan' – Susanne – Stuttgart – Switzerland' do not count (translation Schulz)

With regard to people with cognitive impairments as part of the primary target group of Easy Language, negation can cause problems (Maaß 2015 + Bredel/Maaß 2016). Therefore, the rulebook of the Research Centre for Easy Language recommends avoiding negation or marking it by typographical highlighting to make it more perceptible (ibid.). In the examination of the study which this article relates to, this strategy was applied to spoken language by highlighting negation via intonation. For the avoidance of negation by positive formulations it would appear that the investigator names some examples for words that are allowed after having explained which ones do not count. However, this would falsify the results of the study, which is why the investigator should refrain from it. In the study by Schulz (in preparation) the rules for each part were explained on the basis of another letter with the following remark:

- Wir nehmen jetzt aber einen anderen Buchstaben. Wir nehmen den Buchstaben “P”. Zähle mir bitte Wörter mit “P” auf, die du kennst.

  Let’s take another letter. Let’s take the letter “P”. Please name words starting with “P” (translation Schulz)

However, this requires that the participant is able to retain the rules and apply them to other letters in the tests. It shows that in the conceptualisation of the Regensburg Word Fluency Test, there is still a need to adapt it to people with special communicative needs, in this case, people with cognitive impairments.

3.2 Eyetracking

In the study this article relates to, it was the participants’ task to read texts from the field of health communication e.g. head lice. While reading, the eye movements were recorded by an eyetracking device. The basis for this method is the eye-mind hypothesis according to which the eye movements are related to what attention is focused on and what information is processed (Just/Carpenter 1980). For example, the amount and length of saccades, fixations and regressions allow inferences about the cognitive processes involved in reading. In order for an eyetracking device to record the movements of the eye while reading, the device must detect the pupil first which is ensured in the calibration. The participant should sit 60 to 65 centimetres away from the device and should not move. In addition to the texts themselves, the experiment in the eyetracking program contains instructions that guide the participant through the experiment. For this navigation, whether moving on to the next page should be done by mouse click or by arrow keys can be selected in the settings. The font size within the instruction texts can also be modified, however there are limitations on part of the software which have to be taken into account.

Successful calibration is an important prerequisite for obtaining accurate data for eye movements and reading behaviour. Research shows that drop-out rates in eyetracking examinations with people with impairments are higher because difficulties arise more frequently (see Csakvari/Gyori 2005; Doyle/

Saunders/Little 2016). With regard to people with cognitive impairments Schiffl (2020: 237) states:

> [They] seem to suffer from increased eye deformity, nystagmus and/or squint which impede the calibration process and possibly leads to a loss of quality in the eyetracking data. […] Furthermore, participants of the target group may struggle to restrain their head and body movement, which again is crucial to the quality of eyetracking data.

Based on these findings, the handling of these difficulties in the concrete situation is significant. In order to avoid uncertainty and demotivation on the part of the participant, it is important to turn to him/her, talk to him/her and encourage him/her in case no successful calibration is possible despite several attempts.

Following Schiffl (ibid.), who determines that people with cognitive impairments could have difficulties following the instructions because of impaired concentration and attention span, some adaptations were made in the respective study. In the creation of the experiment, the instruction texts were adapted to the linguistic skills of the target group by means of Easy Language in order to simplify navigation for the participants. Concerning the function to move on to the next page, it has been defined in the settings that the arrow keys are to be used:

> Sie haben den Text fertig gelesen?
> Dann drücken Sie die Pfeiltaste nach rechts.
> You have finished reading the text?
> Then press the right arrow key (translation Schulz)

In this context, a medial strategy (s. chapter 4.3) was also applied: In order to increase perceptibility the arrow keys were provided with green (forward) and red (backward) sticky dots.

3.3 Free Recall

In the study this article relates to, the next step after reading and recording using the eyetracking device was free recall. This means that right after the reception the participant is asked to reproduce as completely as possible what the respective text was about. This can be done orally or in writing (Rickheit/ Strohner 1993: 103). With regard to the cognitive load of people with cognitive impairments, free recall was performed orally by the participants. It was recorded and transcribed afterwards for the analysis.

In the study it was noticeable that the answers given by the participants were initially very brief and that more detailed reproductions were only achieved after repeated encouragement by the investigator.

3.4 Rating

After this unit the participants had to evaluate how well they understood the respective text using a rating scale. A first estimation from the participant can be obtained very easily using this method even if the reliability of the statements given is questionable (Gibson/Levin 1989: 256). Therefore, the data gained by rating should be correlated with that of the other methodological steps.

In the study this article relates to, a four-point scale with the following options was used:

- Ich habe alles verstanden [I understood everything]
- Ich habe das meiste verstanden [I understood most of if]
- Ich habe nicht so viel verstanden [I did not understand very much]
- Ich habe gar nichts verstanden [I did not understand anything]

As the whole examination was conducted as a face-to-face interview (see chapter 3.5), the rating scale was read out to the participants by the investigator with the request to assign comprehension to one of the options. This requires that the participants are able to retain the four options in order to answer appropriately. With regard to people with cognitive impairments as participants, a medial strategy was applied: If the investigator noticed difficulties with answering this question the scale was presented to the participants in print form with enlarged font. The investigator and the participant read the options out loud together and then the participant pointed to the respective one.

3.5 Questionnaire

In the study referred to in this article, a questionnaire was used to collect meta data like age, sex, profession, but also information on reading behaviour, interests and familiarity with Easy and Plain Language. As there is a focus on how well texts are understood and retained by participants with special communicative needs, the questionnaire also contained content-related questions that had to be answered. Following Bortz/Döring (2016: 398) the questionnaire method is characterised by the fact that data is generated in written form.

Filling in a questionnaire independently requires a minimum level of reading and writing skills which de facto excludes a number of target groups, unless questionnaires are adapted to their needs (ibid.). One concrete modification in the study referred to is that semi-structured questionnaires were used and applied in a face-to-face-interview. The whole examination was conducted in Easy Language, audio recorded and transcribed for the analysis. Even though the neuropsychological assessment already provides data with regard to the participants' writing skills, the results are very heterogeneous. Gutermuth (2020: 150) states that in the creation of the questionnaire there should be an orientation towards the weakest in order to establish equal conditions for all participants. As mentioned in 3.3, people with cognitive impairments have limited concentration and attention span in contrast to average participants. That is why the cognitive load of the participants should be taken into account with regard to the extent of the whole questionnaire in order to gain reliable data. Therefore, the number of questions was limited to a maximum of 10 for each text.

4 First conclusions

First research results on content in Easy and Plain Language for people with cognitive impairments as participants lead to the conclusion that current data collection methods require modification with regard to methodology and administration in order to gain reliable data. This results from the specific communicative needs of the target group that have so far not been taken into account properly.

In this chapter the necessary adaptations from chapter 3 are summarized and, in addition, modifications are introduced that concern research with participants with cognitive impairments. The individual adaptations are assigned to linguistic, conceptual and medial strategies. The boundaries of these categories are fluid meaning that a clear distinction is not always possible. That is why the overview is prototypical.

4.1 Linguistic strategies

Linguistic strategies refer to an enhanced perceptibility and comprehensibility of the different oral and written parts in the examination. As mentioned in 3.1 the manuals for the different neuropsychological tests were linguistically adapted to the needs of people with cognitive impairments as well as the language itself during the face-to-face interview. Moreover, at the level of perceptibility, the font size of the instruction texts in the eyetracking software was enlarged. When technical devices are used, however, there may be restrictions concerning these settings which have to be taken into account.

One further adaptation that includes conceptual aspects and is also related to acceptance is that the investigator builds trust in order to create interaction at eye level. In the study referred to, the investigator accompanied the participants from their workplace to the room in which the examination took place. By starting with small talk and introducing the participants to the experiment slowly, a linguistic strategy was applied to help build trust. Furthermore, the investigator tried to sustain the participants' motivation by strategically planning the experiment in advance, knowing the distinct requirements of the target group and the limited attention span (see chapter 3). The investigator encourages the participants to take part in the experiment and explains what their task is. One important aspect in this context is that the participants are informed that they can take breaks during the experiment or even cancel it.

Linguistic adaptations are intended to give the participants a sense of security in the experiment which might represent a stressful exam situation. One example is the simplification of the instruction texts by means of Easy Language in order to avoid complications, mistakes or misunderstanding because of linguistic complexity.

4.2 Conceptual strategies

One important adaptation is the decision where the examination will take place. With regard to ecological validity and ethical considerations, the examination of the study referred to was carried out at the participants' work place which is a familiar environment for them (CRPD 2006: 18, see chapter 1). As mentioned in 4.1 the experiment might be considered as an exam situation by the participants which causes a lot of stress and pressure and cuts off capacities that are actually needed for the examination itself. This was to be counteracted by conducting the experiment in a familiar environment of the participants.

Another conceptual strategy is using semi-structured questionnaires in a face-to-face interview instead of having the participants fill out the questionnaires by themselves. With regard to the cognitive load of the participants, the number of content-related questions in the questionnaire was limited to a maximum of 10 for each text.

In this context, the duration of the whole experiment should also be adapted to the cognitive capacities of people with cognitive impairments. This means that the examination should not be too long, which is even more important when a mixed-methods-approach is applied. Decreasing concentration was communicated by the participants and can be seen in the observation protocol when body posture was noted. Therefore, the participants should be given the possibility to take a break in order to not overstrain the cognitive load.

Furthermore, in the eyetracking part, the keyboard was prepared by means of colour coding (see also Bredel/Maaß 2016) in order to simplify navigation in the software for the participants.

One very important conceptual strategy is to raise awareness of the examination, its research goals and content among the supervisors and staff at the participants' workplace as gatekeepers. This plays a significant role not only before, but also during the entire time of the data gathering process. In the sense of transparency, this is beneficial for the examination itself because disruptions can be avoided (e.g. knocks on the door, confusion when the participant is not at his/her workplace).

Building trust among the participants was already mentioned in 4.1, but can also be assigned to a conceptual strategy. It is important to keep up the participants' motivation and to empower them. This also includes the handling of situations when problems arise which could irritate the participant and give them the feeling that they did something wrong (e.g. in the calibration before eyetracking).

An important conceptual strategy for the investigator and the whole data collection process is to conduct the examination with the help of an assistant. He/she can take notes on observations during the examination in an observation protocol. This could be body language/posture, occurring problems and the participants' reaction for example. These data can be interesting for the analysis in the sense that they are correlated with other results. The observation protocol can be seen as a great relief for the investigator during the examination as cognitive capacity is available for communication with the participants.

4.3 Medial strategies

One of the medial strategies already mentioned in 4.2 relates to the preparation of the keyboard needed in the eyetracking part. In the study referred to, the arrow keys were modified with green (forward) and red (backward) sticky dots in order to simplify navigation for the participants.

In the rating on how well the texts were understood by the participant the medial adaptation refers to its realisation. The scale had an enlarged font and was read out to the participants in the face-to-face interview. When the investigator noticed problems with retaining the four options, she handed out the scale in print form. As a result, the participant could point to the respective option and the investigator marked it with a cross.

Summing this chapter up, linguistic, conceptual and medial strategies (Rink 2020) were applied to adapt the mixed methods in the concrete data collection to the needs of people with cognitive impairments. Depending on the subject these needs can be more or less serious.

The examination itself is often considered as an exam situation by the participants and it is important to decrease the asymmetry during the interaction with the investigator. Furthermore, fears and uncertainties should be prevented and text barriers should be strategically lowered. Thus, the improvement of communication by means of linguistic, conceptual and medial strategies can be achieved “by impacting on communicative action itself or by impacting on the means of communication and therefore indirectly on the communicative action” (Schubert 2009: 110; own translation). It should not be disregarded that contextual factors with regard to the setting of the investigation still needs to be verifiable and controllable in order to have equal conditions for all participants.

5 Conclusion and outlook

Following Rathmann (2020: 2), one reason for not having taken into consideration people with disabilities in general and people with cognitive impairments in particular is that up to now appropriate data collection methods were still lacking. A further reason is that some research disciplines lack awareness with regard to the special (communicative) needs of people with cognitive impairments and other target groups e.g. language learners or children as participants. As participants normally are non-experts there might be certain asymmetries within the test situation or setting that researchers of different disciplines might not be aware of. As barriers, either oral or written, emerge in context it is not the user perspective that has to be taken into account first, but the text perspective (Hansen-Schirra/Maaß 2020). Its according parameters have an influence on the results and therefore have to be modified or rather adapted with regard to the special needs of different target groups.

This paper aims at presenting an approach used in Applied Linguistics and Translation Studies that contributes to appropriate evaluation and data collection methods with regard to the strong communicative needs of vulnerable target groups. Therefore, it can also be considered reliable for these participants (as lay people). In order to allow dependable conclusions regarding the effectiveness of certain issues, it is a necessity for future research to empower cognitively impaired participants by providing accessible texts, content or methods in a first step in order to gain valid results in a second step. From the perspective of applied linguistics and translation studies as well as accessible communication as a new interdisciplinary field of research, the question addressed by this modified approach is: what can be verified by data and evaluation methods that are not understood and/or retained by participants and therefore lead to misunderstanding or incomprehension (see also Rink 2020: 78, 112; Schnotz 1994: 32f.)? If participants do not understand what task they have to perform or what information is given in a text (online, offline, oral or written), then the question is how valid data gained on the basis of helplessness or random answers can be. And, how reliable are these results and to what conclusions do they lead? How comparable is data if it turns out that the linguistic elements used within an examination on the basis of measurable parameters are beyond the necessary prerequisites of the participants?

However, the needs of people with disabilities with regard to accessible health care provision are not well documented. This matters for people with cognitive impairments in a distinctive way: As they have limited reading and writing skills, they are particularly vulnerable and dependent on third parties and their global, grammatical and discourse knowledge. This plays an even more important role when it comes to health issues and health-related decisions. If the health literacy of this group is evaluated, the linguistic elements in the experiment are often above the knowledge level and linguistic skills of non-experts as participants. Furthermore, the subject of the examination itself is often too complex for participants to understand. Therefore, it is necessary that data collection methods are adapted to the needs of people with cognitive impairments. These adaptations include linguistic, conceptual and medial strategies by means of which barriers can be removed from texts and interaction situations. One means to overcome these barriers is Easy and Plain Language that were introduced in chapter 1. Both varieties are mentioned in the National Action Plan Health Literacy as well as in the Convention on the Rights of People With Disabilities in order to provide equal access to information which, in the sense of participation, is a human right.

Literature

Ahrens, Sarah (in preparation): *Patientinnenaufklärung beim Frauenarzt – Welche Eigenschaften müssen Einfache-Sprache-Texte haben, um für Frauen mit Deutsch als Zweitsprache verständlich und handlungsanleitend zu sein?* [Manuskript der Dissertationsschrift, Hildesheim].

Aschenbrenner, Steffen/Tucha, Oliver/Lange, Klaus W. (2000): *RWT – Regensburger Wortflüssigkeits-Test. Handanweisung.* Hogrefe Verlag: Göttingen.

Bock, Bettina M./Lange, Daisy (2017): "Empirische Untersuchungen zu Satz- und Textverstehen bei Menschen mit geistiger Behinderung und funktionalen Analphabeten." In: Bock, Bettina M./Fix, Ulla/Lange, Daisy (eds.): *"Leichte Sprache" im Spiegel theoretischer und angewandter Forschung.* Berlin: Frank & Timme, pp. 253–274.

Bortz, Jürgen/Döring, Nicola (2016): *Forschungsmethoden und Evaluation in den Sozial- und Humanwissenschaften.* Springer-Lehrbuch, Springer-Verlag Berlin Heidelberg.

Bredel, Ursula/Maaß, Christiane (2016): *Leichte Sprache. Theoretische Grundlagen. Orientierung für die Praxis.* Berlin: Dudenverlag.

Bromme, R./Jucks, R./Rambow , R. (2004): "*Experten-Laien-Kommunikation im Wissensmanagement*." https://ams-forschungsnetzwerk.at/downloadpub/experte-laien-kommunikation.pdf (Zugriff: 08.12.2021)

Clark, Herbert (1996): *Using Language.* New York: Cambridge UP.

Csákvári, Judit/Györi, Miklós (2015): "Applicability of standard eyetracking technique in people with intellectual disability: methodological conclusions from a series of studies." In: *Studies in health technology and informatics* (217), pp. 63–70.

Deilen, Silvana (2022): *Optische Gliederung von Komposita in Leichter Sprache: Blickbewegungsstudien zum Einfluss visueller, morphologischer und semantischer Faktoren auf die Verarbeitung deutscher Substantivkomposita.* Berlin: Frank & Timme.

Deutsches Institut für Menschenrechte (2021): *Convention on the Rights of Persons with Disabilities and Optional Protocol.* <https://www.institut-fuer-menschenrechte.de/fileadmin/Redaktion/PDF/DB_Menschenrechtsschutz/CRPD/CRPD_Convention_and_Optional_Protocol.pdf> (Zugriff: 5.12.2021).

Doyle, Lesley/Saunders, Kathryn J./Little, Julie-Anne (2016): "Trying to see, failing to focus: near visual impairment in Down syndrome." In: *Scientific reports* (6), p. 20444. DOI: 10.1038/srep20444.

Flick, Uwe (2011): *Triangulation. Eine Einführung* (3., aktualisierte Auflage). Wiesbaden: VS Verlag für Sozialwissenschaften.

Fornefeld, Barbara (2002): *Einführung in die Geistigbehindertenpädagogik.* München, Basel: Reinhardt.

Geukes, Cornelia (2019): Health literacy und die Konstruktion von Gesundheit und Krankheit aus der Perspektive von älteren Menschen mit geistiger Behinderung. In: *Forum Qualitative Sozialforschung/Forum: Qualitative Social Research*, 20 (2), pp. 1–26.

Gibson, Eleanor J./Levin, Harry (1989): *Die Psychologie des Lesens.* Frankfurt am Main. Fischer Taschenbuch Verlag GmbH.

Gutermuth, Silke (2020): *Leichte Sprache für alle? Eine zielgruppenorientierte Rezeptionsstudie zu Leichter und Einfacher Sprache.* Berlin: Frank & Timme.

Hansen-Schirra, Silvia/Maaß, Christiane (2019): *Translation proper: Kommunikationsbarrieren abbauen.* Uni Hildesheim. https://doi.org/10.25528/015

Häßler, Frank./Eggers, Christian (2012): "Intelligenzminderung". In: Fegert, J.M./Eggers, C./Resch, F. (Hg.): *Psychiatrie und Psychotherapie des Kindes- und Jugendalters.* Springer: Berlin, Heidelberg. pp. 785–833.

Helmstaedter, Christoph/Lendt, Michael/Lux, Silke (2001): *VLMT – Verbaler Lern- und Merkfähigkeitstest.* Göttingen: Beltz Test Gmbh.

Just, M. A./Carpenter, P. A. (1980): "A Theory of Reading: From Eye Fixations to Comprehension." In: *Psychological Review* 87 (4), pp. 329–354.

Keller, Loraine (in preparation): *Verständlichkeitsoptimierte Medizinkommunikation – Akzeptabilität und Akzeptanz von Texten in Einfacher und Leichter Sprache.* [Manuskript der Dissertationsschrift, Hildesheim].

Lehrl, Simone (2018): *Mehrfachwahl-Wortschatz-Intelligenztest: Manual mit Block MWT_B/Siehgried Lehr.* 6. Unveränderte Aufl. Balingen: Spitta GmbH.

Maaß, Christiane (2015): *Leichte Sprache. Das Regelbuch.* Berlin: LIT Verlag.

Maaß, Christiane (2020): *Easy Language – Plain Language – Easy Language Plus. Balancing Comprehensibility and Acceptability.* Berlin: Frank & Timme.

Maaß, Christiane/Rink, Isabel (eds.) (2019): *Handbuch Barrierefreie Kommunikation.* Berlin: Frank & Timme.

Maaß, Christiane/Rink, Isabel (2020): "Scenarios for Easy Language Translation: How to Produce Accessible Content for Users with Diverse Needs." In: Hansen-Schirra, Silvia/Maaß, Christiane (eds.): *Easy Language Research: Text and User Perspectives*. Berlin: Frank & Timme, pp. 41–56.

Petermann, Franz (2008): *Wechsler Intelligence Scale for Adults. Fourth Edition. Manual 1: Grundlagen, Testauswertung und Interpretation*. Frankfurt: Pearson Assessment.

Rathmann, Katharina/Zelfl, Loriane/Kleine, Anna/Dadaczynski, Kevin (2021): *Gesundheitsbewusstsein und Gesundheitskompetenz von Menschen mit Behinderung: Erste Ergebnisse einer Befragung in Leichter Sprache in Einrichtungen der Eingliederungs- und Behindertenhilfe. Prävention und Gesundheitsförderung.*

Rathmann, Katharina/Dadaczynski, Kevin (2020): *Gesundheitskompetenz von Menschen mit Behinderung in Einrichtungen der Eingliederungs- und Behindertenhilfe: Ergebnisse der GeKoMB-Studie (in Schwerer Sprache).*

Ratz, Christoph (2013): "Zur aktuellen Diskussion und Relevanz des erweiterten Lesebegriffs." In: *Empirische Sonderpädagogik* 4, pp. 343–360.

Rickheit, Gert/Strohner, Hans (1993): *Grundlagen der kognitiven Sprachverarbeitung – Modelle, Methoden, Ergebnisse*. In: UTB für Wissenschaft. Tübingen, Basel: Francke.

Rink, Isabel (2020): *Rechtskommunikation und Barrierefreiheit. Zur Übersetzung juristischer Informations- und Interaktionstexte in Leichte Sprache*. Berlin: Frank & Timme.

Rink, Isabel/Maaß, Christiane (2022): "Verständlichkeit und Gesundheitskompetenz im Spektrum zwischen Leichter und Einfacher Sprache". In: Rathmann K./Dadaczynski K./Okan O./Messer M. (eds.): *Gesundheitskompetenz.* Springer Reference Pflege – Therapie – Gesundheit. Springer, Berlin, Heidelberg. https://doi.org/10.1007/978-3-662-62800-3_146-1

Schaeffer, Doris/Hurrelmann, Klaus/Bauer, Ullrich/Kolpatzik, Kai (2018): *Nationaler Aktionsplan Gesundheitskompetenz. Die Gesundheitskompetenz in Deutschland stärken.* Berlin: KomPart 2018 [1. Überarb. Aufl.].

Schaeffer, Doris/Vogt, Dominique/Berens, Eva-Maria/Hurrelmann, Klaus (2016): *Gesundheitskompetenz der Bevölkerung in Deutschland. Ergebnisbericht.* <https://www.uni-bielefeld.de/gesundhw/ag6/downloads/Ergebnisbericht_HLS-GER.pdf> (Zugriff: 5.4.2021).

Schiffl, Laura (2020): "Hierarchies in Lexical Complexity: Do Effects of Word Frequency, Word Length and Repetition Exist for the Visual Word Processing of People with Cognitive Impairments?" In: Hansen-Schirra, Silvia/Maaß, Christiane (eds.): *Easy Language Research: Text and User Perspectives.* Berlin: Frank & Timme.

Schnotz, Wolfgang (1994): *Aufbau von Wissensstrukturen: Untersuchungen zur Kohärenzbildung beim Wissenserwerb mit Texten. Vol. 20.* Weinheim: Beltz.

Schulz, Rebecca (in preparation.): *Medizinkommunikation in Leichter und Einfacher Sprache für Menschen mit kognitiver Beeinträchtigung – eine empirische Studie zum Verstehen und Behalten medizinischer Fachinformationen.* [Manuskript der Dissertationsschrift, Hildesheim].

Schuppener, Saskia/Bock, Bettina M. (2019): "Geistige Behinderung und barrierefreie Kommunikation". In: Maaß, Christiane/Rink, Isabel (eds.): *Handbuch Barrierefreie Kommunikation.* Berlin: Frank & Timme, pp. 221–247.

Seidel, Michael (2013): "Geistige Behinderung, eine Einführung." In: Bienstein, P./Rojahn, J. (eds.): *Selbstverletztendes Verhalten bei Menschen mit geistiger Behinderung. Grundlagen, Diagnostik und Intervention.* Göttingen u.a. Hogrefe, pp. 11–28.

Tischler, Lars/Petermann, Franz (2010): "Testbesprechung Trail Making Test (TMT)." In: *Zeitschrift für Psychiatrie, Psychologie und Psychotherapie* 58 (1), pp. 79–81.

Wimmer, Heinz/Mayringer, Heinz (2019): *Salzburger Lesescreening für die Schulstufen 2–9.* Hogrefe Verlag: Bern.

EASY – PLAIN – ACCESSIBLE

Vol. 1 Isabel Rink: Rechtskommunikation und Barrierefreiheit. Zur Übersetzung juristischer Informations- und Interaktionstexte in Leichte Sprache. 472 pages. ISBN 978-3-7329-0593-5

Vol. 2 Silvia Hansen-Schirra/Christiane Maaß (eds.): Easy Language Research: Text and User Perspectives. 288 pages. ISBN 978-3-7329-0688-8

Vol. 3 Christiane Maaß: Easy Language – Plain Language – Easy Language Plus. Balancing Comprehensibility and Acceptability. 304 pages. ISBN 978-3-7329-0691-8

Vol. 4 Elisa Perego: Accessible Communication: A Cross-country Journey. 200 pages. ISBN 978-3-7329-0654-3

Vol. 5 Silke Gutermuth: Leichte Sprache für alle? Eine zielgruppenorientierte Rezeptionsstudie zu Leichter und Einfacher Sprache. 312 pages. ISBN 978-3-7329-0587-4.

Vol. 6 Anne-Kathrin Gros/Silke Gutermuth/Katharina Oster (Hg.): Leichte Sprache – Empirische und multimodale Perspektiven. 160 pages. ISBN 978-3-7329-0708-3

Vol. 7 Maher Tyfour: Sprachmacht auf engstem Raum: Die Inszenierung der Stadt in den Hörfilmen der Münchner Tatort-Filmserie. Eine korpusgeleitete Studie zur Audiodeskription. 246 pages. ISBN 978-3-7329-0699-4

Vol. 8 Camilla Lindholm/Ulla Vanhatalo (eds.): Handbook of Easy Languages in Europe. 660 pages. ISBN 978-3-7329-0771-7

Vol. 9 Silvia Hansen-Schirra/Katja Abels/Sarah Signer/Christiane Maaß: The Dictionary of Accessible Communication. 212 pages. ISBN 978-3-7329-0729-8

Vol. 10 Katrin Lang: Auffindbarkeit, Wahrnehmbarkeit, Akzeptabilität. Webseiten von Behörden in Leichter Sprache vor dem Hintergrund der rechtlichen Lage. 488 pages ISBN 978-3-7329-0804-2

Frank & Timme

EASY – PLAIN – ACCESSIBLE

Vol. 11 Silvana Deilen: Optische Gliederung von Komposita in Leichter Sprache. Blickbewegungsstudien zum Einfluss visueller, morphologischer und semantischer Faktoren auf die Verarbeitung deutscher Substantivkomposita. 782 pages. ISBN 978-3-7329-0834-9

Vol. 12 Elena Husel: Leichte Sprache in der Bundesverwaltung. Was? Wer? Wie? 250 pages. ISBN 978-3-7329-0849-3

Vol. 13 Sarah Ahrens/Rebecca Schulz/Janina Kröger/Sergio Hernández Garrido/Loraine Keller/Isabel Rink (eds.): Accessibility – Health Literacy – Health Information. Interdisciplinary Approaches to an Emerging Field of Communication. 234 pages. ISBN 978-3-7329-0895-0

Frank & Timme